Dedicated to the memory of Margaret Purss, Harry
Donaghue and Margaret Kelly

Nursing Homeless Men:
A Study of Proactive Intervention

Nursing Homeless Men:
A Study of Proactive Intervention

John Atkinson

PhD, BA, RGN, NDNCert, DipEd, DNT
Senior Lecturer, Adult Nursing, University of Paisley

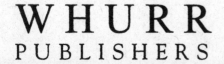

WHURR
PUBLISHERS

© 2000 Whurr Publishers Ltd
First published 2000 by
Whurr Publishers Ltd
19b Compton Terrace
London N1 2UN England, and 325 Chestnut Street,
Philadelphia PA 19106, USA

British Library Cataloguing in Publication Data
A catalogue record for this book is available from the
British Library.

ISBN 186156 149 0

Contents

Foreword

Through innovative and skilful use of both quantitative and qualitative research methods, Dr. Atkinson calls our attention to the medical and caregiving needs of homeless men. This work brings the men and their lives in from the margins. John Atkinson bears witness to the lives of men living in homeless shelters and we are reminded that they belong to us. It challenges mainstream healthcare providers to redraw the boundaries of care. Our common humanity is at stake. We are all injured by those whom we refuse to recognize. This work demonstrates how stereotyping and stigmatization create social invisibility and loss of requisite social skills to access health care.

The nursing interventions are relatively simple and include meeting the men, bearing witness to their plight, and finding out what they perceive their needs to be. Once this is established, they are coached on how to enter mainstream health care. As long as social and health care systems make requirements that marginalized homeless people cannot meet, access to health care is blocked regardless of the number of available health care workers. Atkinson concludes that, with policy and institutional supports, nurses' assessment is an intervention in its own right.

John Atkinson brings himself, as an expert Community Nurse, to this project and demonstrates how the nursing interventions of meeting, establishing trust, coaching and grooming help these men to meet demands required to access mainstream healthcare. Contrary to medical folk wisdom that homeless men are depressed because of their environment, and therefore are unfit candidates for medical treatment, this work demonstrates that only subgroups of the men are depressed. However in those subgroups, severe depression and anxiety freeze the ability of these men to move out of their settings. For these subgroups, medical treatment and social support do help to bring about change.

This rich and provocative study raises many new research questions. The work moves back and forth between explanation and understanding, and in the understanding, John Atkinson brings the men's lives into view. He lays bare the explanatory systems of society and health care providers that explain away the possibilities of care and illustrates that understanding is the bedrock of our common existence.

This book is a must-read for all health care workers. It offers at close hand strategies for beginning where we must, with the felt needs of real persons with real histories. Nursing is particularly well positioned to take up John Atkinson's challenge to meet and bear witness to one another's lives. But, this cannot be done without societal will and vision to redraw the boundaries of our care and connection – this book is a new beginning.

Patricia Benner
Professor of Nursing
University of California

Preface

The study and PhD thesis on which this book is based derived from my earlier work as a generic district nurse with a special interest in the care of homeless men (Atkinson 1987). Having secured a Scottish Office Nursing Research Training Fellowship and subsequently further funding from the Scottish Office Health Service and Public Health Research Committee, a full-time research study was initiated.

The main objectives of the study were to present health profiles of the residents of a hostel in Glasgow and a comparison hostel in order to make assessments and referrals, and to evaluate their effect. These objectives were successfully met, along with the secondary objective of discovering insights into the residents' experiences and lifestyles, and their interaction with health and nursing services. The objectives were addressed by gathering and analysing quantitative and qualitative data, and by the use of theoretical perspectives: Roy's (1980) nursing theory of adaptation (to study the men as individuals) and a sociological perspective, including deviancy theory, to examine the men as a group. Recommendations regarding health and nursing care policy and practice for this client group were also made.

Two hostels for homeless men in Glasgow — the Great Eastern Hotel (Main Study Hostel) and the James Duncan Hostel (Comparison Hostel) — were used. Employing a questionnaire of 26 questions, validated tools (the Barthel Index of physical function, and the Hospital Anxiety and Depression Scale) and an alcohol use questionnaire, the study described the hostels and undertook health and lifestyle profiles of the residents. One hundred and six residents were interviewed in the Main Study Hostel (by the project nurse) and 100 in the Comparison Hostel (by the researcher).

In the Main Study Hostel, John Dreghorn, the project nurse, undertook nursing assessments of the sample he interviewed. Interventions were then made: immediate treatments; referrals to health professionals (who were subsequently interviewed to evaluate their responses) and acts of advocacy. Sixty-six men received district nursing interventions, which included 9 types of treatment, 11 of referral and 17 of advocacy.

Six sample referrals to district nurses were presented to an expert panel of district nurses for comparison. Significant levels of physical and psychiatric morbidity were found, including possibly treatable biogenic depression. The data suggest that some of this may not be caused by being homeless but occurs beforehand. Significant differences in practice patterns were demonstrated between district nursing using a case-finding approach and district nursing reacting to specific referral.

Although the study concentrated on district nursing practice, it demonstrated universal methods of nursing practice relevant to all community nurses, in particular targeted case-finding for homeless people and other groups of marginalized clients, using its assessment, referral and monitoring techniques and methods of recording quantitative and qualitative data.

This book will take the reader through the study, its results and the insights made. To ensure that the book is as readable as possible, some of the intricate detail of the study's results has been omitted or summarized, and an emphasis has been placed on explanation. I am very happy, however, to provide readers with details of the work and thesis (Atkinson 1997) on application.

The study became the basis for a PhD thesis. The work was, therefore, written up in a strictly logical fashion in order to enable the design, method, findings and analysis to be exemplified with clarity. As the reader may imagine, given the nature of the subject matter, the study, from its inception, did not run on straight rails. The book will highlight features of the sometimes winding journey taken by the study, in order to assist practitioners and future researchers in their endeavours.

Finally, it is hoped that readers, particularly nurses, will be encouraged to undertake their own work, large or small, with the assurance that, although some areas of nursing are difficult, all areas benefit from systematic examination. Patient care can be improved when the patient is considered both as part of a group in a specific context and as an individual.

Acknowledgements

I would like to thank the following people:

- John Dreghorn, the project nurse, whose contribution made the study so fruitful, and whose wit and quiet humour saved many bad days;
- Glasgow District Council Homeless Unit, Hamish Allen Centre, Glasgow for access to the Comparison Hostel;
- the owner and staff of the Great Eastern Hotel, Glasgow;
- Glasgow Council for the Single Homeless;
- Professor David Walsh and the Department of Social Sciences, Glasgow Caledonian University;
- Mr Mike Shewry, Glasgow Caledonian University, for tutelage regarding the computer statistical package;
- Dr R.P. Snaith, Consultant Psychiatrist, St James's University Hospital Leeds, who acted as expert witness with regard to the anxiety and depression score results;
- Ms Marion Miller, librarian, Glasgow Caledonian University;
- the Greater Glasgow Health Board Community and Mental Health Unit for permitting the project nurse to practise as a district nurse.

On a more personal note, I am indebted to my two nursing supervisors, Professor Margaret Alexander and Professor Jean McIntosh, and to other members of the Department of Nursing and Community Health, Glasgow Caledonian University, for their generosity and persistence, and to my sociology supervisor, Mr Des McNulty, for his encouragement and stimulation.

To all of these special thanks are due, particularly to Margaret and Jean. I was, and remain, a thoroughly bad-tempered student at times, and the often painful personal journey that this study entailed meant that they were witness to those disagreeable parts of my personality I usually try to keep hidden.

Various contacts were made with other professionals outside Glasgow by letter, telephone and visit. These included nurses working in similar areas, for example Barbara Stilwell, an internationally respected nurse practitioner who works with homeless men in London (Stilwell and Stern 1989); Stilwell and her colleagues had worked with men in hostel-type accommodation. Also contacted was Dr L.McAndrew, an author in Edinburgh who provided information on the mass assessment of physical function (McAndrew and Hanley 1988).

Thanks go too to my two external examiners, Professor Tony Butterworth and Professor Fiona Ross. Both made very helpful suggestions for the completion of the original thesis.

I would also like to acknowledge the help and support of my family and friends, particularly my wife Patricia and children Eilidh and Iain: family and social life was held in abeyance on several occasions. Thanks also to my former employer Mr Roger Houchin, Governor, HM Prison Barlinnie, where I was Health Centre Manager. At the time I was trying to finish my thesis, Eilidh and Iain were 2 and 1 years old; it became impossible to achieve anything at home, and I thought I would never finish. Roger gave me perission to be locked into my office at night for several week-long periods in order to allow me to finish.

Finally, thanks go to my present colleagues, particularly Mr Jack Rae and Mrs Liz Kennedy at the Department of Nursing, Midwifery and Health Care, University of Paisley where I am a Senior Lecturer, for their help and support.

Chapter 1

Introduction

Study background

> Following the dictates of his heart, he has deliberately taken the victims' side and tried to share with his fellow-citizens the only certitudes they have in common – love, exile and suffering. (Albert Camus, *The Plague*)

This study is about a group of single homeless men, their lives and experience, particularly their interaction with health and nursing services. It is also about the doctors and nurses who provided care for them and the difficulties they encountered. The study attempts to provide insight into the men's experience and the attitudes and working practices of the doctors and nurses. Recommendations are made for future practice.

In 1984, the author moved from London to Glasgow to begin working in Glasgow's East End as a qualified district nurse with two general practitioner (GP) practices. These two GP practices were located in the largest health centre in Glasgow.

The East End of Glasgow was an area of mixed housing, mainly council owned, with sections of relative affluence and employment but also deprivation and unemployment. There were several light industrial sites, but the old, mainly heavy, industries associated with the area, for example Parkhead Forge, had gone. During the 1960s and 70s, many of the old tenements and closely packed streets of shops had disappeared, and some high-rise flats had been built.

During the 1980s, a large regeneration programme was undertaken with new housing schemes (some on old industrial sites), including special housing for the elderly and disabled. The effect of this work was to completely change the profile of the area, with the dismemberment of the previous tight communities, many associated with particular industries and religious groupings (Protestants and Catholics drawn mainly from the North of Ireland since the nineteenth century).

By the end of the 1980s, some of the housing had become owner occupied, but the area was still predominantly working class. The health centre mentioned above was built as part of the regeneration, combining several small practices that had been based in the various communities.

Having come from a multiethnic and multicultural area of London, the author was particularly aware at the time of how many of his colleagues came from the east of the city and of the ethnic homogeneity of the area.

The development of the author's interest in the homeless

In the geographical area of the health centre, several hostels for homeless men existed. In particular, there were two large commercial establishments that had been there for many years. There was also a night shelter run by the Church of Scotland (in an old kirk) and a hostel organized by the Salvation Army. In addition, there were three council-run hostels, which had been built in more recent years. The presence of these establishments meant that there was an obvious (even to a casual observer) presence of often old, dishevelled men walking about the streets.

Not long after he started work at the health centre, the author was approached by a district nurse colleague who ran clinics for homeless men at a nearby shelter and asked whether he would be interested to work with her in this field. The author started working in these clinics two afternoons a week as an extended part of his normal GP practice-attached duties. The work consisted of offering first aid, wound care and the administration of some medications prescribed by one of the GPs from the health centre, who took a special interest in the men. The district nurse colleague subsequently left the area, and the author continued alone.

The clinics served a useful purpose. Men who would otherwise not receive care were provided with a basic service that, on occasion, prevented a further deterioration in their health and circumstances. They also received individual care and kindness. The author kept an informal record of all these contacts. Over 100 individuals attended, of whom 30 were considered 'regular' clients.

The clinics were limited in their scope of practice and possible long-term beneficial effects because even the more regular visitors attended only sporadically and only when they were in extreme need. Others would come for a wound dressing, for example, but not return for many weeks. Further men would be seen opportunistically on the street or met in tenement close doorways (apartment stairwells).

The author, as a district nurse, did not feel that he was entering or influencing the men's lives and experiences in a meaningful way. The clinics, while useful, appeared to have no context. The nurse and his 'patients' appeared to meet and pass almost as ships in the night. The work was entirely reactive and dependent on the men making contact with the district nurse at the clinic. As an example of the author's dependence on the men approaching him, one individual returned to see him after over 2 months – still wearing the same leg bandage. As a nurse, the author felt some pride at the efficacy of his bandaging skills and the fact that no lasting damage had occurred. However, it did demonstrate that this was a limited pattern of practice.

The author decided to make professional visits to where the men lived and make contact with them there, hopefully on a more regular basis. This 'proactive' approach might, he thought, enable the service to become a more integral part of the men's lives and also give the author a clearer insight into some of the core health and social problems that the men experienced, possibly enabling him to influence these in a positive way.

Gaining access – main problems discovered

To begin with, the author had great difficulty gaining access to the commercial hostels. As with any other form of accommodation, health professionals have no automatic right of access, and the hostel management showed hostility towards the author. The Glasgow Council and Church-run establishments were, however, agreeable to access.

Having gained access to the largest hostels, the author found that one of the main health-related problems that men faced was that many were not registered with a doctor, and they often did not have their hostel as their registered address. This state of affairs meant that, bureaucratically speaking, they almost 'did not exist' for the purposes of gaining social service benefits and receiving health care.

During the next 3 or so years, the author, along with others in the regional social work unit and the Glasgow Council homeless unit, assisted men to register with a GP and to access mainstream health services. This had a profound effect on many of the men who received relevant care for the first time. The author reported this work in an article (Atkinson 1987). The following advantages and disadvantages were recognized. In health terms, having a registered address and a GP enabled many of the men to be seen by a doctor on a regular basis. This gave them access to primary, secondary and tertiary care. It also enabled them, when relevant, to receive medical examinations and supporting letters to housing and other agencies.

It would be incorrect to overemphasize the success of this work. The homeless men still met with many difficulties, even if they were registered with a GP. A degree of prejudice was shown by health professionals, particularly related to the men's real or assumed alcohol consumption and their inability to live in normal accommodation. Also expressed by many health professionals was a reluctance, as they put it, to 'waste precious resources'.

Although the author, as an advocate and interested agent, appeared to assist initiate beneficial effects for some of the men, there appeared to be many unanswered questions. First, was there a role for the district nurse with this specific group, namely single homeless men? Everyone seemed to admire the work from a moral point of view in that it was a 'good' or 'right' thing to do. This was, to be honest, quite beguiling in that the author felt worthwhile and valued, but it was difficult to describe the processes and exact function of the nurse – what difference did the work make?

Second, there was very little in-depth research regarding the health care of single homeless men that could provide an insight into some of the practical and professional difficulties that nurses faced when working with patients in this group. These factors made the author think, 'Well, something will have to be done. What about me?' It was important, he thought, for someone to take the issue of the health care of homeless men very seriously and for the area of work to be accepted as worthwhile for advanced nursing practice and research.

The author gained funding as a Scottish Home and Health Department (now the Scottish Office Department of Health) Nursing Research Training Fellow and commenced the preparation for the study. In 1992, further funding was awarded to continue the research, the main aim of which was:

> To assess the health and nursing needs of a group of homeless men and to evaluate a system of referral and of district nursing intervention designed to meet the identified needs.

This book is, therefore, the manifestation of a 12-year professional, academic and personal journey.

The Industrial City of Glasgow – a brief historical background

The problems of single homeless men in Glasgow cannot be properly examined without referral to the history of Glasgow's industry, working population and demographic patterns, housing policy and homeless provision.

'The Clyde made Glasgow and Glasgow made the Clyde' is a commonly heard adage. It refers to the fact that although, like many other great cities, Glasgow is built along the banks of a river, the River Clyde was systematically widened and deepened over two centuries to accommodate the industry and transport needs of the emerging Industrial Revolution. This symbiotic relationship lasted until after World War II. The growth of the city was accompanied by immigration and population moves from the mid-eighteenth century onwards, particularly from the Highlands and Ireland (Hamilton 1981).

Eighteenth century

The writer Daniel Defoe visited Glasgow in 1727 and described the emerging city and population, with Glasgow's wide streets and busy life. These streets and the green spaces were, in the main, built in a spacious and orderly manner to cater for the population of this busy port, with its interest in the tobacco industry (Defoe 1753).

Nineteenth century

With the Industrial Revolution, the next 150 years saw the population grow from a few thousand to 1 million (slightly larger than its present size). Industry was varied: tobacco, textiles, foundries and ship-building all had their role. During this time, the pressure on housing became immense, the demand outstripping the supply. Connected with this pressure were the concomitant problems for the working population's health and welfare brought on by conditions in the factories and other workplaces and exacerbated by overcrowded housing, poor nutrition and the inadequate and sometimes dangerous water supply (Douglas 1987).

The types of work available created openings for a large number of transient male workers. The combination of overcrowding, bad health and the need to house transient workers was experienced by many port cities during this time.

From the mid-nineteenth century into the twentieth century, local government, religious and voluntary organizations and commercial operators became involved in providing shelter, regulating housing and providing pastoral care to these workers.

Housing

Tenements were classified by the number limitation of their residents: small plaques, placed on the wall of the building, stated the number of people allowed to live there. Adherence to these regulations was at best variable, at worst ignored altogether (Checkland and Lamb 1982, Greater Glasgow Health Board, personal communication, 1993). For single men, hostels were available. To overcome overcrowding in these establishments and the exploitation of the residents, so-called 'model' lodging houses were set up. These provided men with a cubicle or partitioned space for single occupancy, as well as certain basic hygiene facilities.

From working man to single homeless

Twentieth century

During the earlier part of this century, several organizations and employers provided hostel-type accommodation for single men. The provision tended to be similar to the old 'model' system, although the commercial establishments were usually called 'working men's hotels'. Glaswegians tended to (and still do) call all these places 'models'. They had an ambivalent attitude towards them. On the one hand, many working people had unmarried male relatives and other people they knew living in hostels; working men from differing backgrounds would go for their lunch at some of the larger hostels. On the other hand, these establishments developed a name for drunken and disorderly behaviour and were identified with the seamier side of Glasgow life. The names of these hostels became locally notorious.

After World War II, the industrial base of Glasgow's employment began to diminish, the opportunities for temporary, transient and manual labour becoming fewer in number. Glasgow is today almost unrecognizable in comparison with its past. In the North West of the City, Springburn's rail workshops are no more. In the East, Parkhead Forge, where huge naval guns were produced – the sound of its giant hammers being heard throughout the area – has been replaced by a supermarket complex. To the South, where the river bank was once covered with shipyards creating every kind of floating vessel from small launches (many of which were used in the Dunkirk evacuation) to the QE2, there is now only one shipyard on the Clyde. These industries used to employ tens of thousands of men each (Smart 1988).

The East end of the City of Glasgow was a predominantly working-class, industrial area. The hostels are therefore predominantly centred around this area. During the 1970s and 80s, the clientele of the single men's hostels was seen to change (Glasgow Council for Single Homeless 1984). Many of the men who had lived in the hostels became unemployed, and the hostel population aged. Their lifestyle and physical deterioration was mirrored by the deterioration of the fabric of the buildings. Men who had become homeless for other reasons were also becoming residents (Glasgow Council for Single Homeless 1984, Atkinson 1987).

The hostels and working men's hotels became associated with homelessness. Today, the norm is that only a very small proportion of hostel residents are in paid employment. During the 1970s, Glasgow District Council (GDC) built a number of hostels to cater for homeless men. They were built with single rooms instead of cubicles, but the communal washing and eating facilities remained (Glasgow District Council Information Unit, personal communication, 1992).

Glasgow hostel accommodation

Council provision

The GDC provides hostel accommodation for about 1100 men and 150–200 women. Not all single homeless people are accommodated in hostels, although a significant proportion are (Glasgow Council for Single Homeless 1990a).

Night shelters

The voluntary sector, for example the Talbot Association, provides indoor space (known as 'night shelter') for those who sleep rough. The Salvation Army had until recently a hostel for 90 men, although this is now closed. The Church of Scotland has a building that used to be a night shelter but which has now been registered as a residential home, still for homeless men. This provision is typical of many large cities (Garside et al 1990).

Private hostels

Three hostels in Glasgow are privately owned. The Bellgrove normally has approximately 80 residents, the Monteith approximately 29 residents. These two hostels have largely stable populations with little resident turnover. The Great Eastern Hotel formerly had space for 500 residents, but the usual number of residents is now between 120 and 200.

The term 'hostel' is used by statutory and voluntary services to describe the type of accommodation available to single homeless men, although private establishments are often titled 'hotels'. The establishments used in the study will be called 'hostels'.

Services

Glasgow has an integrated system of provision for single homeless people; that is, hostel-dwellers have access, at the time they register and beyond, to assessment by and action on the part of the GDC Homeless Team and the Social Services Homeless Team, who attempt to place residents in suitable accommodation.

This integrated system has been brought about by the GDC Housing Department, Strathclyde Regional Council and the Glasgow Council for Single Homeless (GCSH), which comprises members from all the statutory and voluntary bodies and also provides a housing project for young homeless people (Calderwood 1989, Glasgow Council for Single Homeless 1989a, 1989b, Glasgow District Council and Shelter 1991). The combination of these bodies has produced an ongoing multidisciplinary strategy. This has resulted in target-setting and evaluation. Targets include the setting up of alternative accommodation and the reduction of the need for night shelter services (Glasgow Council for Single Homeless 1984, 1989b, 1989c, 1990b, 1991).

In conclusion, this chapter has described the author's early work as a district nurse with single homeless men and how and why he became interested in the need for, and to carry out, detailed research with this group. The chapter has also given a brief background history of Glasgow and the statutory and voluntary provision for homeless men in the city, in order to provide the context in which the study is set. The author thus set up a study describing and evaluating district nursing intervention with the residents of the largest commercially run hostel for single homeless men.

The next chapter will present a review of the literature that informed the author on the definitions of and wider issues regarding homelessness, other projects with homeless men and philosophical aspects of health care provision in the UK and other Western countries that affect the care of homeless and marginalized people. It will also present the theoretical framework of the study. The study of these areas enabled the author to formulate the aims of the study, together with the design and method.

The reader may already be able to observe how many different strands of knowledge, history, practice and policy are coming together in an attempt to answer what appears to be a relatively simple set of questions, for example 'Does nursing these homeless men do any good?'

This complexity will be seen to stem from two main features. First, there was no precise definition of homelessness, associated ill-health or what practitioners were supposed to do about it. Second, and most importantly, as the study began to scratch the surface of the literature, both theoretical and fieldwork, nothing was as obvious as it first appeared. These two themes run throughout this book.

Chapter 2
Literature review

Introduction

This chapter presents a review of the literature. The reader will observe the complexity and length of the review, and it is important to clarify the reasons for this. First, it became apparent from the start that the terms used by professionals working in the area meant different things to different people, the term 'homelessness' being the best example. Second, in order to instigate a rigorous study, it was important to explore and make explicit all the potential areas of enquiry that the study would undertake so that the design, fieldwork, findings and analysis could all be undertaken using a consistent and solid base of knowledge. The review thus has four distinct but connected sections that will take the reader through the various elements of the study:

1. Definitions, descriptions and measurements of the occurrence of homelessness are given, along with the effects both on health and within the policy-making context.
2. Having established these effects, a critique of five reported projects on delivering health and nursing services to homeless people provides further background to this study and leads to a discussion of the literature pertaining to the generic role of the district nurse and the possibilities for a specific role with homeless people.
3. During the examination of project reports and other literature, evidence was found that the attitudes, assumptions and beliefs held by health professionals, homeless people and society as a whole appeared to influence the amount and nature of the care provided and received. The third area, therefore, considers some of the philosophical aspects that underpin health-care provision and influence health professionals' views of their work, exemplifying these aspects with examples from the literature.

4. Progressing from this discussion comes the study's theoretical framework, which highlights the individual's adaptation to health-threatening stimuli (using Roy's nursing theory; Roy 1980) and a sociological view (including deviancy theory) that emphasizes the men as a group, responding to one another as well as to health-care providers and society.

Limitations of the literature review

It is important to point out at this stage the limitations of the literature review, particularly as an introduction to a research study. At the beginning of the study, many articles, reports, government policy documents and descriptions from voluntary agencies about homelessness in general and single homeless men in particular were examined. This wide-ranging search proved extremely useful in the assessment of the range of practice, definitions of homelessness and its associated health problems, as well as in illustrating how this study might proceed. Statutory and voluntary agencies highlighted priorities for action. There were very few dedicated research studies addressing the assessment of and intervention for health need with groups of homeless people, that is, where individuals designed and conducted a study, made planned interventions and evaluated their effects.

However, there were a number of the reports, particularly in the UK, describing the range of medical conditions that health professionals identified among the homeless. The reports describe the care and treatment given and the clinical evaluations of the services that were made. Others describe homeless patients, particularly the mentally ill, and their impact on health services. These clinical evaluations provided important background detail and influenced the choice of the type of intervention and method of practice appropriate for this study.

Five clinical evaluation projects regarding health-care provision and single homeless people are described in detail. The projects described contained an element of nursing practice, although they were not written from a nursing perspective. No published nursing research projects were discovered before the setting up of the study, even though the author was in contact with nurses who worked with homeless people. One nurse was studying rough sleepers but not from a nursing perspective and had not published at the time. Although there was a lack of specific nursing research, the literature review nevertheless provided a strong foundation for the study.

Nature and method of critique of the literature review

Having established the limitations of the literature, it is important to highlight how value was allocated to the wide variety of articles, reports and other literature examined.

As will be demonstrated, there were few precise definitions of terms such as 'homeless'. In addition, some of the literature demonstrated an interesting approach to data collection and access to sample groups, for example, but did not reach any major conclusions or relate the findings to the projects' stated aims. In the five critiques, these anomalies will be demonstrated, including, in one, the use of a district nurse as a data collector but not as a practising nurse.

Other literature, particularly that from various political and voluntary pressure groups, made assertions and recommendations without necessarily demonstrating clear causal links or a rationale. It had to be decided whether to limit the literature review to the examination of research or to seek information and insight from as wide a base as possible; the latter approach was chosen. However, it is important to state that equal value was not placed on all items of information gathered.

The method used to design the study was to read the various items of literature and highlight the key points. As the author's knowledge increased, certain key features emerged either by their regular occurrence or by being referred to in several sources. Other features became noteworthy because they referred particularly to the study's sample group, that is, homeless men. By a process of reflective analysis, assimilating some features and rejecting others, the design and method of the study gradually took on a structured and logical form.

Definitions and implications of homelessness

The home as a social concept is strongly linked with a notion of family – the parental home, the marital home, the ancestral home. The word 'home' conjures up such images as personal warmth, comfort, stability and security, it carries a meaning beyond the simple notion of a shelter. (Watson and Austerberry 1986, p 8)

This quotation illustrates how there is no absolute definition of homelessness. In terms of this study, this is an important place to start as it requires the setting out of the study's fundamental terms of reference. There appears to be agreement in the literature that homelessness does not just mean roofless or shelterless (Watson and Austerberry 1986); that is, people may have a roof over their head and still be homeless.

In recent years, therefore, the term 'homeless accommodation' has emerged. This is a recognition that some individuals, although they have shelter, do not have a home (Victoria Community Health Council 1984, Wooton 1985). Shelter, the national voluntary organization for the homeless, and other organizations such as Crisis, recognize the definition of home quoted above and tend to define homelessness in terms of people who do not have a permanent domestic base, who are without a recognizable social context and who lack other human requirements:

> security, privacy, sufficient space, a place where people can grow and make choices ... Vandalism, graffiti, fear of violence, lack of play space, all affect how people regard their surroundings. How property is managed, as well as its physical condition is important as it affects how people make decisions. To believe that you have no control over one of the most basic areas of your life is to feel devalued. (Shelter 1991)

An important feature of this statement is its objective and subjective elements, that is, that homelessness involves a lack of certain amenities and physical necessities, but also includes an individual's perception of his or her state. As will be demonstrated later, particularly in Chapter 8, individuals' views of their circumstances directly relate to their physical and social experience.

Another feature of the above statement is that it describes the elements that are important to consider with regard to where all people live, placing homelessness and homeless accommodation on a continuum of living conditions with other accommodation. In later chapters, it will be seen how some individuals in the study regarded their hostel as 'home' whereas others did not. The statement, however, also demonstrates the difficulty, for this study, in defining exact terms of reference for the word 'homeless'.

Defining who is homeless – the statutory duty and policy context

To address the difficulties in defining the term 'homeless', the literature from government agencies was examined. Central government collects statistics from local authorities, who have a legal obligation to house families with children (called 'households'), pregnant women, the elderly, the disabled and other vulnerable persons under the terms of the the 1977 Housing (Homeless Persons) Act and the Housing Act 1985 (Part III). Local authorities record households who report as homeless and are provided with temporary, and then more permanent, accommodation. The effect of the emphasis on data collection from homeless households is that government and voluntary services' statistics are dominated by data about families. Nearly 70% of homeless people recorded are children (Shelter 1988, Thomas 1991).

The term 'single homeless' has been used since the mid-1960s to describe unattached (i.e. having no partner or family) hostel-dwellers and those sleeping rough (Powell 1987a). The terms 'sleeping rough' and 'skippering' are used to refer to people who sleep outside in temporary shelters (e.g. cardboard boxes) or in buildings not designed as dwelling places (such as derelict premises). In the literature these individuals are often referred to as 'rough sleepers'. 'Squatter' is the term used to refer to individuals who take over empty dwelling properties and set up home.

Local authorities do not have an obligation to house the single homeless, rough sleepers or squatters unless they fall into the Housing Act categories, so the number of single homeless people is not recorded centrally. Estimates vary, the Campaign for Homeless and Rootless (CHAR) suggesting that there may be 2 million single people in the UK who are homeless (Shelter 1991).

Difficulties in quantifying the problem

Having stated some of the definitions of homelessness, any attempt to discover the extent of homelessness is a confusing process. Estimates of the size of the homeless population depend upon the group or agency that is used as the source of information. The lack of a central collation of statistics is one problem, and, as has been described, this combines with the tendency of statutory agencies to collect statistics only on those homeless people *for whom they are responsible*.

From a health-provision standpoint, this poses a problem, given that health agencies usually have a general remit to provide care for everybody in their area. Macmillan et al (1992), when setting up their survey in Glasgow, describe this dilemma – Greater Glasgow Health Board having a remit of care provision for everybody within its geographical boundaries, whereas the Glasgow City Housing Department's responsibility is to its citizens or residents.

Homeless people are seen in town and country, although local authority experience has demonstrated that they are mainly seen in towns (Bonnerjea and Lawton 1987, Department of the Environment 1987, Courtney 1988). Accommodation for the homeless, such as hostels and bed and breakfast hotels, is found mainly in cities. This has led to the geographical displacement of people from the surrounding semi-rural and rural areas.

For example, the GDC does not place its homeless citizens in bed and breakfast hotels. It has a centre (the Hamish Allen Centre) where homeless people report and are assessed, and there is a variety of emergency accommodation that is used, in the first instance, before individuals or families are accommodated in mainstream housing. However, the surrounding local authorities, for example Paisley and Falkirk, place homeless persons in bed and breakfast hotels in Glasgow's geographical area (Glasgow District Council, Hamish Allen Centre, personal communication, 1992). Thus, there are actually in the city many hundreds of homeless people living in bed and breakfast hotels, the number of those in bed and breakfast accommodation in Glasgow being unknown.

Classification of homeless groups and individuals

Rough sleepers

It has been observed that the most obvious homeless, those sleeping in cardboard boxes for example, are often not recorded as homeless (Shelter 1990a). On the night of the 1991 census (21–22 April) 2703 people were found sleeping rough (outside with no roof) on 453 sites in the UK. Shelter estimates that 20 000 people sleep rough from time to time in the UK, about 8000 in a single night (Shelter 1991, Keyes and Kennedy 1992). It should be emphasized that these are estimates and, apart from the Census, have not emanated from a systematic 'head' count.

Families

Families, with children under 16, may be classed as 'unintentionally' or 'intentionally' homeless. The former often occurs when families living in someone else's home have to move out when the situation becomes intolerable for both parties. Intentional homelessness often also happens after a family has been offered accommodation and has refused it. For example, a woman who has been physically abused and has become homeless may refuse to go back to a house in the area where she suffered violence (Murie 1988, Shelter 1988).

To present the most accurate number of homeless families or 'households' is difficult. However, 126 680 households were accepted as being unintentionally homeless by local authorities in the UK (Shelter

1991); Shelter have estimated that this may constitute 363 300 individuals.

Homeless families may be placed in bed and breakfast hotels as a temporary measure. Many, especially the intentionally homeless, gravitate to illegal multioccupancy flats where there will be a family living in each room of a flat designed for one family (Brimacombe 1987, Atkinson and Thompson 1989, Shelter 1990b).

The Health Visitors' Association and the General Medical Services Committee (1989) described the situation thus: 'More than 100,000 families are estimated to have no permanent home and are forced to occupy various types of temporary, often sub-standard, accommodation.' It is important to highlight, in a research study, the prevalence of estimated numbers used in all the literature available on homeless families and individuals. This lack of precision regarding the size of homeless groups became an ever-present feature of the current study of the literature.

Young people

Young people registered as homeless when they are 16 are classed as 'young single homeless' until they are 25 years old. An increase in the number comprising this group has been seen over recent years. This has been associated with changes in benefits for young people since April 1988, when young people between 16 and 18 were disallowed from receiving benefits (Gosling 1989). Among these are young people in child care; some have been in a homeless state for some time before they are 16 (Gosling 1990, Glasgow Council for Single Homeless 1989a). Again, these assertions must be regarded with some care as no empirical link has been made between the 1988 benefit changes and youth homelessness; there is merely a suggestion that the changes had a complicating effect for already vulnerable individuals.

Single homeless people

Single homeless people are those living in hostels or sleeping rough. Most single homeless people live in hostels or other designated homeless accommodation. There are many more men (estimated at 90% of the single homeless) than women (Garside et al 1990). With reference to single homeless men, there are similarly no official statistics. Figures available suggest that they may make up about 7% of the homeless total (Shelter 1988), but this figure is likely to be inaccurate as there is no central collation of either those who sleep rough or those staying in hostel provision. Furthermore, the exact number of hostels in Britain is unknown (Berthoud and Casey 1988).

In their postal survey of hostels, Berthoud and Casey (1988) found that there was a large number of hostels for ex-offenders. An often-quoted number regarding the single homeless is taken from CHAR, who estimate that there may be 2 million single homeless people in Britain (Shelter 1991). This figure is not based on detailed research and must therefore be considered with care, especially as it suggests that approximately 1 in 30 people in Britain are homeless.

From the London Housing Unit, examining hostel accommodation, and the organization Single Homeless in London (SHIL), estimates for London of 65 000 single homeless people and 3000 sleeping rough have been made (Single Homeless in London 1987, Shelter 1991). The methods of data collection in these cases are more rigorous as they are based on postal surveys, visits to voluntary agencies and day centres, and the collation of information directly from the providers of residential accommodation. These figures compare with an approximate figure of 300 000 single homeless people in London if the CHAR estimate is correct. Extrapolating these London findings to a national level, as some estimates do, is probably, however, misleading.

A further problem exists, in terms of a research study, in that most of the available literature that presents estimates of the number of single homeless is produced by organizations that provide political advocacy for this group. Thus, whereas the baseline number of families accepted as homeless by local authorities mentioned above is available to compare with the extrapolated estimate of individuals made by Shelter (1991), no similar baseline government information is available for comparison regarding the single homeless. To summarise, in terms of policy-making and service delivery, single homeless people do not exist as a discrete group requiring specific government provision. Their number is therefore neither centrally measured nor known.

National profile of hostel residents – the 'typical' resident

National profiles of all types of hostel, including those for mothers and babies, women's refuge and young people, show the hostel population as being young to middle-aged, mainly in mixed hostels, with more women than men in single-sex hostels. In general, very few hostels specifically provide for those over retirement age, although some elderly men stay in hostels (Berthoud and Casey 1988). The view that the hostel population is young to middle-aged is misleading when considering single homeless men and looking at the large hostels (with populations of over 100) and the age range of residents (Drake et al 1981). Garside et al's (1990) sample was of non-specialist hostels in Manchester, Bristol, Birmingham, Westminster and Lewisham, where most of the bed spaces were for men.

It will be seen from this description that the number of single homeless men is not known with any precision. Most studies cited collected their data by establishing the number of beds available in hostels and their designated purpose. No evidence was discovered of the systematic tracking of groups of identified individuals. This process would have given a clearer picture of the dynamics of the groups, including the relative transience or permanence of the group and from where the hostel residents had originated in the wider community.

Having stated this limitation, the broad profile described above is paralleled in other countries, particularly North America. In summary, what emerges is that if a homeless person is middle-aged to elderly, with no family and in medium- to long-term accommodation, that person is most likely to be a man (Daly 1989, Drake et al 1989, Onyett 1989, Simon Community 1989).

The effects of homelessness on health – an overview

The remainder of this section will describe the connections found in the literature between homelessness and health. This information has come from a variety of sources, including project reports and clinical evaluations of health carers working with homeless people. A more detailed critique of five of these reports will be made below. The purpose of this description is to demonstrate the variety of physical and psychiatric morbidity identified in the literature, which will place the five project descriptions in the next section into context.

Historically, a connection between homelessness and housing conditions such as overcrowding has been demonstrated in the literature. Measures taken by previous generations to combat overcrowding, such as the 'model' lodging hostels discussed in Chapter 1, have emerged today as homeless accommodation (World Health Organization 1989). Living in homeless accommodation has been reported to have a detrimental effect on individuals trying to access more secure accommodation and employment (Gosling 1989). In addition, people living in homeless accommodation often demonstrate signs of poor physical and psychiatric morbidity (Quick 1990).

Within the past 10 years, the significance of health in housing and homelessness has received media and professional attention. Health professionals from many disciplines have recognized the relevance of their skills, particularly in assessment, treatment and referral. The increase in community care, particularly of psychiatric patients, has raised political and professional awareness (Anderson 1984, Lamb and Talbot 1986, Timms and Fry 1989, Ambrosio 1991).

The government policy of promoting and increasing the home ownership of council housing and its effect on the housing stock available has been cited as affecting the health of those who cannot take advantage of the home ownership schemes. In particular, people with special needs (ethnic minorities and the mentally ill or people with learning difficulties) and/or poor health have difficulty gaining access to housing (Single Homeless in London 1987, Wall 1991).

It should be stated, however, that the literature does not present precise causal links between the policy of home ownership and the difficulties encountered by people with special needs; it is presented in the literature more as a political argument than as a fact. The problem could be considered as a lack of service flexibility rather than a direct effect of policy. However, as the 'pool' of rented housing stock has diminished, flexibility in meeting the needs of individuals with special needs has been reduced (Association of Community Health Councils 1989). People with special needs and/or poor health may thus be more at risk of becoming homeless.

Health and single homeless men

Owing to the statutory responsibility of local authorities and health services to provide for homeless families, it has been argued that there is a service emphasis on this group (Health Visitors' Association and General Medical Services Committee 1989). This emphasis may be more easily understood in the context of the legal obligations of child surveillance and welfare having an important role in health professionals' work (Lovell 1986). In contrast, single homeless people are seen as autonomous citizens for whom statutory responsibility is limited.

Williams and Allen's (1989) study, which is discussed below, showed that particular conditions and disease patterns are more commonly found in single homeless men. Mental illness is the best recognized in the literature, in particular by Barry et al (1991), in their overview of current knowledge on homelessness and health. There is considerable mention in the literature regarding the delivery of mental health services. Psychiatrists and community psychiatric nurses (CPNs) in particular are described as delivering care to homeless people both as part of their normal duties and also through special initiatives. Hamid and McCarthy (1989) describe a special community psychiatric nursing service for the homeless in London. Particular emphasis is placed on the care of those who have been in long-term psychiatric hospitals.

Physical illness is also a common feature among the homeless (Williams and Allen 1989), the effects of cold weather and overcrowding on physical health being described. Crisis (1992) describe government action to provide funds to voluntary organizations specifically to provide warmth and prevent hypothermia. Malnutrition among the homeless is described in an American study in which the authors found that homeless people had no regular place where they could get nutritious food (Hales and Magnus 1991).

In the UK, the lack of a food 'outlet', combined with an irregular lifestyle pattern, is seen to be one cause of single homeless people's, particularly men's, malnourished state (Williams and Allen 1989). The exacerbation of 'common ailments' such as chest infections and gastric disturbances, as well as acute serious illness, is described by Park (1989).

Infestation is commonly seen (Atkinson 1987), and pulmonary tuberculosis is also encountered. Substance abuse, particularly of alcohol, is often presumed to be at the root of the health problems the men experience (Keyes and Kennedy 1992). Physical morbidity is associated with factors such as sleep deprivation, loss of privacy, social isolation, trauma and loss of occupation (Park 1989). Certainly, a picture emerges of the harsh physical circumstances of homelessness having a devastating, precipitate effect on health.

A significant number of homeless men spend time in prison. Combined with mental illness or impairment, poor physical health and subsequent discharge back to homeless accommodation, these men often present with multiple health problems combining physical and psychiatric morbidity (Brimacombe 1990, McMillan 1991).

One of the most significant groups of homeless men is that of the elderly. Over a period of 10 months, one nurse, in a limited study, visited 30 elderly homeless people in London who were sleeping rough or in hostels. She found physical and psychiatric illness. Some of the homeless wanted to remain where they were. Others wanted permanent housing but no longer had the physical or psychological ability or strength to do anything about their situation; they were trapped (Crane 1990).

Crane (1990) and others (Wake 1991, Shanks and Smith 1992) have also recognized the ageing effect of homelessness. Many homeless people demonstrate clinical signs usually associated with people over 60 at a much earlier age. These include dementia, physical frailty and early death. Thus, the term 'elderly' may be used to describe a homeless person in, for example, his fifties.

Anecdotal evidence suggests that the state of being homeless is itself hazardous to health (Crane 1990). These descriptions generally emanate not from a purely empirical base, that is, one with objective indicators, but from the experience of those working with homeless people who have observed the appearance and frailty of individuals. However, as the homeless people described in the literature often have a variety of other problems, including poverty, substance abuse and malnutrition, it would be difficult to assert that homelessness was by itself a direct cause of the premature ageing, but truer to say that it compounded any problems that the individual had. It has been estimated that between the years 2001 and 2027, 22.5% of the population will be over 60–65, and the number of elderly people who are in poor housing or who are homeless will have increased significantly from its current level (Leather and Kirk 1991).

Psychiatric morbidity

Some of the elderly homeless have been long-term patients in psychiatric hospitals, and many of these individuals do not have the living skills necessary to manage in a sophisticated social context. Lamb and Talbot (1986) in the USA stated that individuals had been made homeless often not simply because they had been discharged from hospital, but because of the way in which their discharge was achieved, that is, how well the individuals were prepared for discharge and what arrangements were made for their ongoing support and social networking.

This is supported by evidence from the UK, where discharge policy has been adapted in some areas, particularly in multiagency liaison between hospital and community, and specific accommodation provided for the ex-patients of psychiatric hospitals (Anderson 1984, Lamb and Talbot 1986, Medical Campaign Project 1990a, Kelling et al 1991). The Medical Campaign Project (MCP; 1990a), a lobbying group for the homeless, published guidelines for the discharge of the mentally ill from hospital that included the need to establish a firm social context for patients and highlighted the danger of their becoming homeless if their domestic and social environment collapsed.

Hollander and Hepplewhite (1990), in the UK, highlight the lack of housing options and community services for the mentally ill. Reflecting the MCP guidelines mentioned above, the main problem cited is that not enough attention is given to providing patients with supported care, the emphasis instead being placed on medication and supervision. The literature cited here is not research based: it is based on the experience of those who have been involved in the discharge of patients from long-term hospitals (Lamb and Talbot 1986) and those who have to provide care for patients in the community (Hollander and Hepplewhite 1990). In terms of this study, it is recognized that the care of discharged long-stay patients in hostels may be an issue, but the study is not based on that premise.

Differentiating between health and social problems

Identifying the difference between health and social problems has been acknowledged as problematic (Metters and Department of Health 1991). The chronic nature of many homeless people's health problems exacerbates difficulties in their social circumstances and vice versa (Bayliss and Logan 1987). Clapham (1991) describes how the 'policy prescription' for these problems is non-specific 'community care'.

More recent legislation, investigation and literature emanating from the NHS and Community Care Act 1990 has highlighted the difficulties that service providers encounter when attempting to meet the needs of groups in the community, including the homeless, particularly in the definition of what exactly constitutes 'health' and 'social' care. A lack of practical definitions leads to practice and budgetary 'shunting', in which the responsibilty for individuals and groups is denied by health or social service providers because they do not precisely meet their criteria (Ross 1993, Goss and Kent 1995).

Metters (Metters and Department of Health 1991), then Deputy Chief Medical Officer at the Department of Health, describes the single homeless man as the 'paradigm of the homeless person'. Supporting this statement, he observes that such men are seen by health professionals as difficult to care for and hard to reach, thus making systems of care hard to effect.

These difficulties have led to central government pressure to provide for this group. The Department of Health and Social Security circular (1985) directed family practitioners to plan services for the single homeless. Hospital discharge and after-care, together with inter-professional liaison, were recognized as key areas for improvement and action (Yeudall 1988, Barry et al 1991, Lowry 1991).

Summary

In their discussion paper based on a study of the current literature and knowledge on homelessness and health, Barry et al (1991, p7) state that there is 'a broad range of physical illnesses related to the condition of homelessness'. The literature review for this study has thus concurred with this view as well as with their recognition that homeless people suffer from two other groups of health problems: alcohol- and drug-related, and psychiatric conditions (Barry et al 1991).

Health-care projects with homeless people: the role of the nurse

The previous section provided definitions of homelessness and the main groups of homeless people, including single homeless men. This section will examine in more detail the literature, particularly evaluations, pertaining to the delivery of health care to single homeless men. Following this examination, the function of the district nurse and his or her possible specific role with single homeless men will be highlighted. The purpose of this section is to demonstrate the factors that influenced the practical method and research design of the study. The section will conclude with a presentation of some of the conceptual aspects and difficulties encountered and described by other writers, this presentation forming the link with the following section. First, however, a short critique will be presented of studies that have evaluated the work of five health delivery projects for homeless people in London, Bristol and Edinburgh.

Project 1 – Health care for single homeless people

A mainly descriptive study into the health needs of single homeless people was carried out by Williams and Allen (1989) from the Policy Studies Institute in London. The study evaluated two projects in London that provided care for single homeless people. Both were staffed with multidisciplinary teams and were specifically set up as experimental pilot studies with a view to providing a model for future practice.

Sample, tools and method

During 1987, information was collected about the users of the two pilot projects that had an integrated records system. The first scheme, in the City and East London, gave care to 885 individuals during the year, the second, in Camden and Islington, to 576 individuals. The City scheme's multidisciplinary team comprised a doctor, a CPN and an alcohol counsellor; the second was composed of a doctor, a nurse and a project co-ordinator.

A cohort of 190 homeless people were interviewed about their health and lifestyle. Fifty per cent of them had used the pilot projects. Of the 190 homeless people, 90% were men and 10% women. All of the multidisciplinary staff in the project were interviewed, as were a sample of other health-care professionals (34 GPs and 42 district nurses, CPNs and social workers) in addition to voluntary agency members and the wardens of various hostels who also delivered statutory services to homeless people.

Findings

The homeless – those who used the pilot projects

The study described some of the difficulties that the sample of homeless people encountered. These included gaining access to services and GPs refusing to take them onto their lists. High levels of physical morbidity were recorded, particularly respiratory and gastrointestinal complaints. Two-thirds of the sample said they had wanted to see a doctor during the previous year. A so-called 'inappropriate' use of accident and emergency (A and E) departments was highlighted by health-care professionals, contrasting with the men's expressed difficulties in getting care. The concept of an 'inappropriate' use of services will be revisited below.

No preference was shown by the homeless people between attending a special clinic or attending a GP practice, although they expressed frustration if a doctor was not available. A third of the pilot scheme users said that they would try to use an A and E department if the project were not there. The rest were not confident about getting appropriate care or else stated that they would not bother to seek medical attention.

The carers

The carers involved with the pilot projects were critical of mainstream service providers for being inflexible. Two-thirds of the statutory and voluntary providers interviewed thought that homeless people needed dedicated primary health-care services, although there was a realization that this could isolate the patients. Stress was placed on the way in which social and health problems were often inextricably linked and difficult to address.

While recognizing that the success of the pilot projects could not be judged merely on the basis of the number of people who used them, the study team also recognized that a problem of interpretation existed; that is, if one of the aims of the pilot projects was to encourage people to use mainstream services, a high number of homeless people attending the pilot project clinics might be considered to be an indication of failure. This illustrated one of the management problems encountered by the pilot projects, namely that precise operational objectives in terms of the multidisciplinary team and its dealings with the patients, other agencies and their definitions of success had not been made explicit. Although the City pilot scheme saw 885 people and made 3198 consultations, and the Camden scheme 576 people in 2022 consultations (a high proportion being for alcohol abuse and mental health problems), the study team had difficulty in determining success because it was difficult to measure direct links between interventions made by the service and successful clinical outcomes.

Main recommendation

The main recommendation from the study of the pilot projects was that local GPs should integrate the clinics into their mainstream practice rather than that the pilot projects be continued in their present form (i.e. with salaried GPs). Also recommended was that there should be more detailed research into the health needs of homeless people, particularly those who did not use services.

Discussion

The main difficulty for the pilot projects appeared to be that although the teams set up their service in an appropriate location – near a large number of homeless people – and certainly saw many patients, they acted as independent professionals treating a number of homeless people on an individual basis. There were no project and team objectives and outcomes that would be considered a success in terms of the project rather than just in terms of their own professional success indicators with each individual. If the project's objectives had emphasized improvement and an increase of access and health input, success could have been more clearly defined.

Project 2 – Audit of work at a medical centre for the homeless over one year

This report, by Toon et al (1987), was an evaluation of a voluntary evening centre for the single homeless in the City of London run by doctors, nurses, a chiropodist and social workers. The audit ran from February 1982 to January 1983.

Sample, tools and method

Two hundred and sixty-six people, of whom 13 were women, were seen. Most were aged between 40 and 45 years. Individuals were examined on a 'walk-in' basis, and their health status was recorded under the following medical categories: gastrointestinal; central nervous system; ear, nose and throat; obstetrics and gynaecology; dental; skin; respiratory; traumatic; psychiatric; and alcohol. Hospital referrals and outcomes were recorded, as were chiropody consultations. A nurse volunteer was sometimes available. Her input was not recorded separately but is described as acting as 'a receptionist and nurse'.

Findings

Forty-three per cent of the sample had no fixed address, 36% providing a hostel addresses. Forty-seven per cent were registered with a GP. The project estimated that fewer than 40% of the whole sample had 'reasonable access' to general NHS medical services.

Forty-three per cent received a detailed examination from the GPs. Of this subgroup, 33% had alcohol problems, 17.5% pulmonary tuberculosis and 33% a psychiatric history. Seventeen and a half per cent had a history of fractures and 10% one of peptic ulceration. Burns, infestation and head injuries were also seen. The prevalence of the morbidity described was considered to be higher than in normal general practice.

Seventy of the sample were referred to a hospital consultant, a letter being given to the individual and one sent to the hospital consultant. Forty-one consultants wrote back to the project team. Of the 41 individuals on whom the consultants reported, 29 did not take up their appointments, 5 attended once and 2 were admitted but subsequently defaulted. Five completed their hospital treatment.

Main recommendations

The main recommendations were that although expected problems, such as alcoholism, were seen, it was important not to adopt a stereotypical view of the homeless, as a great variety of other physical and psychiatric conditions were also seen. What are often considered minor ailments in general practice, for example injuries and infections, can cause homeless people great problems. The main problem identified was that homeless people lacked the facilities to tend to their ailments and also to maintain general, protective good health.

In the project report, the dilemma posed by the specialist treatment of the homeless was discussed. Specifically, it was stated in the report that if health professionals accept that, as a basic human right, everyone should have access to health care, there should be no need for specialist services. The drive should instead be to educate health professionals to be more tolerant towards this patient group and to treat individuals with more understanding, taking into account the difficult circumstances in which they live. The report concluded that this option was unrealistic as many of the problems, such as a poor uptake of referrals, emanated from the homeless individual's suspicion of mainstream bureaucracy. The provision of specialist services that were more approachable seemed a better option. The report suggested that there was a need for centres similar to the project centre, as well as that some GP practices should take a special interest in the homeless, making them welcome and integrating their care into the mainstream.

Discussion

This project did not attempt to be representational of the homeless population, reporting only on those who used its services. Interesting insights were, however, gained. As in the Williams and Allen (1989) study, a difficulty in measuring success solely on the basis of the outcome of medical examination and referral was described. There was a strong reference, however, to the need for access to services (which was desirable and acceptable to homeless people) as an aim and performance indicator in its own right. The report also highlighted the dilemma of specialist service versus mainstream care as being 'unrealistic', recommending a midway approach in which the specialist service assists the individual into mainstream care.

The project demonstrated similarities with the author's early experience of providing a clinic, described in Chapter 1, with the notable exception that the individuals' problems were described in medical terms at the outset, with no formal recognition of a clear nursing role despite a nurse being available on occasion. The project offered no insight, therefore, into the nursing care of homeless people.

Project 3 – A mobile surgery for single homeless people in London

El Kabir et al (1989) set up the above project in 1987 and gained funding from the London–Edinburgh Trust to purchase a van, equipped as a mobile surgery, to care for rough sleepers at two sites in inner London. It was manned by a doctor and two health professionals (medical students or other health workers). The aims of the project were to discover and describe 'the social and medical characteristics' of the homeless people as well as the acceptability of this form of medical facility. Each site was visited weekly. The study at the first site ran from October 1987 to June 1988, and the study at the second site from June 1988 for 3 months.

Sample, tools and method

A standard questionnaire was used to collect data and form a written assessment of the homeless individuals. Some treatment was given to the homeless people on site. As with the previous project, the individuals' health status was recorded under the following categories: gastrointestinal; central nervous system; ear, nose and throat; obstetrics and gynaecology; dental; skin; respiratory; traumatic; psychiatric; and alcohol. Referrals were made to a nearby medical centre (where there was an inpatient 'sick bay' facility) or other primary health-care sites. For secondary or other care, individuals were recommended to attend mainstream health centres for further treatment or referral; that is, no formal referrals were made.

Findings

Sixty-one individuals were seen on the first site in 121 consultations; 85 were seen on the second site in 123 consultations. The data were considered 'highly similar' and were therefore combined. Of the 146 patients, 13 were women. The mean age of the sample was 40 years (range 16–64 years). Ninety-five per cent of the sample were receiving social security payments, and 17 individuals claimed to have work. One-third of the sample claimed that they never used homeless accommodation. Sixty-two per cent did not have a GP.

Traumatic injury was seen in 15 cases, two complicated by osteomyelitis. Five cases of pulmonary tuberculosis, 15 of bronchitis and 11 of chronic obstructive airways disease, as well as epilepsy and peptic ulcers, were also recorded. Alcohol-related illness was recorded in 10% of cases.

As with the previous project, a suspicion and mistrust of mainstream health services was expressed by many of those who attended, which dissuaded them from seeking help for sometimes serious ailments. Ten people were admitted to the sick bay, and of these, four went on to take up permanent housing.

Main recommendations

The project, that is, the provision of this form of mobile facility, was considered to be a success, particularly as an acceptable access route for homeless people to medical care and the further use of this type of facility were recommended within that context.

Discussion

In this project, ease of access to medical care was made a primary aim and success indicator. The other aim was to provide a social and medical description of the individuals. This was also judged to be successful. However, it is difficult to see exactly what purpose the collection of the medical data had for the individuals concerned. No referral system was organized to primary or secondary health-care sources: further care appeared to depend on recommending the individual to attend a GP. Given the low uptake rate of referrals recorded in the previous project (Toon et al 1987), this being cited by El Kabir et al (1989), it may be mooted that the likelihood of success of referral could be expected to be poor.

A logical conclusion might have been to question the efficacy of expending great effort in creating a system of referral in order for it to fail. It is far better, it could be argued, to keep the process to simple verbal advice that might have a similar outcome (i.e. the uptake of secondary care) and therefore be judged to have the same level of success with the minimum of effort.

As this and the previous project involved medical services, they concentrated on the alleviation of the effects of morbidity. Given the living environment of the samples, however, the projects were limited as the project professionals did not intervene or interact with the individuals' context; that is, they addressed homelessness not as an entity but only in terms of its medical manifestations. This limitation raised conceptual questions that will be discussed below in the section examining some of the philosophical underpinning of health-care systems.

Project 4 – Health surveillance project among single homeless men in Bristol

In terms of the study described in this book, Featherstone and Ashmore's (1988) project in Bristol was important for several reasons. The aim of the project was to undertake a systematic health surveillance of a sample of single homeless men resident in inner-city hostel accommodation. The health checks were carried out by a district nurse and had been instigated following a health centre-based report that found, in 1985, that a number of its homeless male patients had pulmonary tuberculosis. This led to the organization of the surveillance project in two hostels. One was a modern, well-appointed hostel, the other a sparsely furnished 'squalid' residence.

Sample, tools and method

The two hostels catered for 150 men, of whom 91 had been resident for 3 or more months. These provided the sample for the project. Thirty men were already registered with the practice, 10 men were on the lists of other practices who gave access to the project team, and 51 men were not registered at all. All 91 of these men were invited to join the practice.

A questionnaire and examination were administered by the district nurse. A battery of laboratory tests of blood and urinalysis were also carried out. Chest X-rays were offered to all the subjects. Other investigations were carried out when clinically indicated. The data were collected in individual survey casebooks and then read and examined by two doctors. Where there was any doubt, a second opinion was sought from another GP. The casebooks then became part of the patients' medical records. Referrals were followed through by the project team and their uptake measured.

Findings

At the start of the project, some difficulty was experienced as hostel workers told the men that the surveillance was a mandatory health check. The district nurse had to overcome this problem by working with the men and explaining the precise nature of the study.

Of the sample, 51 (56%) had a full medical examination. A variety of conditions were discovered, and 18 were found not to have a significant medical problem. As in other projects, respiratory-related diseases were recorded. Problems associated with the use of alcohol were discovered in nearly half the men. Eighteen men had a history of psychiatric illness or were presently receiving intervention; the project did not appear to seek out undiagnosed psychiatric morbidity.

Social factors were described in broad terms. Forty-one of the men were unemployed, 21 had 'financial difficulties', 8 were claiming sickness benefit, and 6 had 'family problems'.

Main recommendations

The project reported on its success in gaining access to these men, whom it asserted were 'itinerant' and 'disorganized'. It emphasized the success of action by the district nurse, who, after the project was completed, continued to visit the hostels. The main recommendation was to set up peripatetic surveillance in hostels and other places used by homeless people, with the purpose of integrating their needs and treatment into mainstream primary care, emphasizing the model of the project as being 'cheap and easy'.

Discussion

Although this project employed a district nurse, the emphasis, as in the other projects, was on describing morbidity. Whereas some of the conditions described were medically specific, for example 'rapid atrial fibrillation', others were described so generally that it was difficult to ascertain how a diagnosis, for example, 'Twenty-five men (49%) were alcoholics', was achieved.

Again, the emphasis was on clinical manifestation as opposed to how health and illness affected the life experience of the individual men. It was not possible to judge whether there was any relationship between their physical and mental state and their homeless condition. For example, was their illness preventing them from taking other opportunities for an improved lifestyle and better health? This was particularly the case in the surveillance of mental illness, which centred around past history or men already receiving treatment, as opposed to discovering the present psychological state of distress or well-being, which may influence an individual's daily actions.

Similarly, social 'problems' were not examined in a systematic way apart from categorizing large groups under labels such as 'unemployed'. The sample were termed 'itinerant', yet, in order to provide a stable sample, the sample had been selected from men who had been resident in the hostels for 3 or more months.

The fact that the district nurse was asked by the men to return was the only indication given that they found the project helpful or relevant. There was no indication of the nursing role, that of ongoing monitoring and care, and its part in the prospective peripatetic service. The nurse's primary function appears to have been as a data collector for this medical surveillance project. Having cited these difficulties and possible shortcomings, the project did, however, provide a broad model for the study in that it showed that systematic interviews had been achieved in hostel settings similar to those in Glasgow and by a district nurse.

Project 5 – The Edinburgh primary health care scheme for single homeless hostel-dwellers

Powell's (1987b, 1988) study reported on a project in Edinburgh that had originally started 10 years earlier. The project had been initiated in the first instance not because homeless people had difficulty in obtaining primary health care if they wished it, but because concern had been raised with the Health Board that single homeless people were using A and E departments 'inappropriately', that is, attending departments with ailments that should properly be seen by a GP (Powell 1987a). As a response to this 'apparent failure of the single homeless to use the normal procedures' (Powell 1987b, p445), it was decided to regularize access to GPs by utilizing the regulations pertaining to working men's camps, which appoint 'house doctors' to particular establishments and pay them a capitation fee for the number of residents rather than for the individuals registered to their practice.

This project was of particular interest for this study because it was based in Edinburgh, the second largest Scottish city after Glasgow, in a cluster of hostels around the city centre area of Grassmarket, being of a configuration similar to that of the Glasgow hostel scene. The project also involved a district nurse and a health visitor.

Sample, tools and method

During one week in July 1985, 547 single homeless hostel-dwellers were identified from all the hostels and an age/sex register was constructed that formed the basis of a sampling frame. Structured interviews were then carried out with 157 single homeless people, the hostel managers, GPs in the locality and doctors from the local A and E department. The interviews were carried out by 12 medical students and a research assistant. Financial inducements for the residents were discussed but rejected, citing Shanks (1981; also cited in the previous project reports), who demonstrated evidence that the consistency and accuracy of interviews with hostel residents were dependent on the interviewee knowing the interviewer, and that residents were hostile to authority figures. Registration records were also examined at the Health Board to ascertain any previous knowledge of residents and their past medical histories.

Findings

The incidence of physical and psychiatric morbidity was very similar to that described in the projects examined above, with high levels of psychiatric disorder, epilepsy, chest and gastrointestinal disease and alcoholism. The residents expressed general satisfaction with the project, although women (22 being interviewed) preferred to be seen by a female GP. The 15 managers were similarly satisfied, although the site of the central clinic (in an old environmental health disinfestation unit) was considered stigmatizing.

Both groups saw the GP as the best first point of contact, although the district nurse and the health visitor were very welcome. The hospital doctors recognized the benefits of reducing inappropriate referrals and also of a point of contact for outward referral. Powell (1987a) also found that residents using the project used the A and E more appropriately than those who did not. The four GPs, the district nurse, the health visitor and the Health Board administrator were also pleased with the project, considering it to be an appropriate response to this patient group.

Some disadvantages were, however, recognized, many to do with the payment of GPs and provision of GP cover. It was also acknowledged that there was no access to half of the residents' past medical records, resulting in the situation that, for these people, any meaningful health monitoring could only take place after they became residents at the hostel (when they became the house doctor's patients).

Main recommendations

The main recommendation addressed this last point, that is, that modifications should be made to integrate the residents' care and medical records' administration into normal primary health-care practice rather than transient workmen's camp provision. Better facilities were sought, as were a better psychiatric and social work liaison and service.

Discussion

Powell's (1987b) study of this project provided useful markers for the current study, in particular in the use of interviews for the residents and practitioners, and the confirmation that, if asked in an appropriate manner, residents appeared to be as co-operative towards research as did any other group in the general population.

Complicated access-gaining devices and financial incentives were not needed. Again, as in the other project reports, a description of the role and function of the nurse was virtually absent apart from peripheral reference to it. In common with the other reports, there was a concentration on describing how the homeless people's problems impinged on the health services rather than how health and illness affected the homeless. In the case of Powell's (1987b) project, this was probably influenced by the reason for the initiation of the project – to regularize the residents' 'misuse' of A and E departments.

Lessons for the current study from the five projects examined

The following important lessons for setting up the current study were learned from an examination of these five project evaluations:

1. A combination of the quantitative measurement of needs and personal, demographic and social factors with a record of interventions, along with qualitative interviews of the homeless men and their care providers, provided a more holistic description of the homeless people and the problems faced in delivering care to them.
2. The aims and objectives of the proposed study should emphasize input of intervention and increased access to care as measures of success.
3. The proposed study should include a general health profile that would be useful with regard to the care of the individual as well as

providing an insight into the health of the group. It might be difficult precisely to describe success in every individual case, but the
information gained would assist the whole group.
4. The proposed study should describe the residents' experience of their
health and lifestyle rather than just how these factors impinged on
health services.

Entering into the patient's experience

The five projects described above, and other work found in the literature, demonstrated that the treatment of morbidity is only one element
of the delivery of care to this client group. Some projects reported
'success' when staff engaged with the men as individuals. They
concerned themselves with clients' quality of life and everyday
existence, providing small personal services, entering into their experience and gaining insight into how the men perceived their life and
health.

Stern and Stilwell (1989), as a GP and nurse partnership, provided
clinics for homeless men incorporating a wide variety of treatment,
social and referral possibilities. Burke Masters (1988), a nurse working
single-handedly in a clinic for homeless men, acted as her patients'
friend and advocate as well as treating physical conditions. Donaghue
(1989), a Red Cross worker in Glasgow, set up a bathing service for
elderly men in the Main Study Hostel (Glasgow Council for Single
Homeless 1991). Many of the homeless people described in these
projects benefited from medical care. Where it was present, they also
gained from nursing care.

Dant and Deacon (1989) remark that the rehabilitation of the
homeless is not simply a matter of providing suitable housing and
practical assistance but of helping individuals to adjust and professionals to respond to their clients' needs from a tolerant and multifac-
eted perspective.

The district nurse

The formalization of nursing in the home and community, provided by
professionals, emerged in the 1850s. In 1887, the women of Britain
presented money for Queen Victoria's Golden Jubilee, this money
being used to form the Queen's Nursing Institute. This organization
formalized district nursing by providing premises, training and professional structure on a national basis (Baly 1987).

As has been described earlier, the effects of 'bad' housing arising
from circumstances of overcrowding, poor sanitation, communicable

diseases and financial poverty have long been recognized, particularly by health professionals. From their inception, district nurses have been involved in the care of people in poor housing and those who are homeless. Flora Lees, one of the first district nurses, writing in her diary at the end of the nineteenth century, describes her encounters with 'recalcitrant' landlords when trying to get better conditions for her patients (Baly 1987).

Until the 1970s, district nurses tended to work in geographical areas. In town and country, the nurse became a well-recognized member of the community, sometimes occupying a particular house in a village or town. During the 1970s, 'primary health-care teams' were instigated. The basic principle of these teams was to provide care within a GP's caseload from district nurses, health visitors, social workers and midwives who were attached to the practice (McIntosh 1985). This remains the norm today, although there are still geographically based nurses, particularly in cities, where GP practices overlap.

Acheson (1981) also recognizd that primary health-care teams work well in areas where the population is stable and registered with a GP. Practice-attached community nurses are not formally responsible for the whole of their community but only for the patients of the practice. Thus, in cities, unregistered and transient people are frequently missed, and homeless people have found doctors and nurses unwilling to register them (Heuston et al 1989, Stilwell and Stern 1989).

GPs', and increasingly district nurses', work is mainly reactive and caseload restricted: the patient must seek out the doctor, who then refers him or her to the district nurse. Neither GP nor district nurse tends to treat patients outside the practice. This structure somewhat restricts the nurse's potential to act. Other impediments to a broader practice base described for district nurses are a rigid learning structure, badly informed management and low political status (McIntosh 1985, Mackenzie 1992). These factors may make it difficult for district nurses to provide innovative care for groups who fall outside the GP's practice.

Types of service available

District nurses have, therefore, found their present role restricted despite the historical connection of practice with the poor and homeless described above. Most referrals come from the medical profession, and the possibilities for autonomous case-finding are seldom fully explored (Badger et al 1988a). This restricted role is contrary to the education and professional background of many district nurses, which emphasizes the importance of social study and autonomous networking.

District nurses can be effective practitioners with groups of the poor and homeless. They are commonly experienced clinical practitioners with a knowledge of social policy, the health services, statutory benefits, health promotion and communication skills, and accustomed to delivering care in varied and often difficult environments with limited resources and 'back-up' (Baly 1981, Atkinson 1989).

Reactive versus proactive practice

With their education and training, and clinical and community work background, district nurses may be seen as suitably qualified to work in a professional capacity with single homeless men. It is important to highlight areas of difficulty; that is, does anything prevent district nurses delivering an effective service to this group? This happens despite recommendations that the homeless need imaginative proactive health care (Brickner 1986).

Barriers to practice

The main drawback to broader-based practice, including the care of the homeless, centres around the fact that the district nurse receives most of his or her caseload reactively from medical referrals. Badger et al (1988b, p 1362) recognize this factor thus:

> The scientific medical model permeates our health care system. Not only are nurses squeezed into a restricted outlook, geared more to health problems than to individuals with health problems, but they also tend to view patients in isolation from their social situation.

The author's own experience as a district nurse working with homeless people supports this statement. His early work in hostels tended to be seen as unofficial, much of it having to be achieved in lunch breaks. The management view was often that the work was distracting him from the treatment of his caseload. Referrals are often based around a medical diagnosis, and the district nurse's visiting pattern tends to emulate that of the GP. The nurse visits a patient to undertake a particular procedure in a limited time, rather than visiting the patient and and spending some time not associated with a particular pathology. This time is where an appreciation of the patient's whole perception and experience may be gained.

Audit and unrecorded activity

Some audit systems used in the health services to monitor district nursing and other health-related services may also hinder practice because of insufficient information (Badger et al 1988a). These systems often equate efficiency with the number of procedures undertaken rather than with any value added to the patient's quality of life (Peterken 1990, Hart 1991). The more qualitative aspects of professional work may go unrecognized and therefore not be valued. Qualitative intervention or monitoring is often not recorded and therefore not included in analyses. At the time of the study, for example, the work-recording forms used by district nurses in Glasgow merely enabled the nurse to record treatments (e.g. dressings) and baths given.

Status of nursing in the homeless care field

Johnson and Challis (1983) observe that an antimedical 'lobby' is present among some social services working in the community, as a result of an attempt to get away from medical dominance. In their view, this has resulted in patients being deprived of medical and nursing services. Certainly, in setting up this study, it was found that nurses' status among other professionals working with the homeless was not high. It would, however, be a mistake to labour this point. No direct evidence, either in the literature or in the study, was found of systematic antipathy on the part of other professionals in the homeless field towards medical or nursing practice. Taylor (1992), examining discharge from psychiatric hospital into the community, also found prejudicial attitudes in nurses, suggesting that 'vagrants' have brought their condition on themselves and are thus to be treated with less tolerance.

So whereas there is a group of health professionals with the skills to address the care of single homeless people, namely district nurses, a combination of referral and practice patterns, possible attitudes and assumptions (on the part of the nurses and other professionals) may create barriers to effective delivery. These possible barriers and attitudes led in this study to the examination of some of the conceptual and philosophical underpinnings of the medical and nursing professions to see whether they brought any insight into the difficulties in delivery of care and the attitudes shown towards the men.

Philosophical aspects

This section will briefly examine and discuss some of the underlying philosophies that inform and direct health-care provision in the UK and other Western countries. It must be emphasized that it does not provide a philosophical critique in the classical sense; that is, this section will not provide a discourse on philosophical propositions or follow their logic through a series of questions and conditions to 'prove' their relative value. The section will instead be restricted merely to highlighting the presence of philosophical concepts and assumptions, with examples from the literature, in the decision-making of health professionals, particularly in relation to their consideration of whether individuals should receive care and how the appropriateness and level of intervention of that care to the individual and certain groups, particularly the homeless, should be decided.

Reducing problems into treatable parts – the Cartesian approach

So far, this chapter has attempted to demonstrate how homeless people are a group of individuals demonstrating complex physical and psychiatric morbidity within an often dysfunctional social context. Some of the literature, particularly from the USA, begins to explore the possibility of whether 'homeless' can be defined as a recognized illness or condition. Park (1989) describes this complexity as the 'etiology of homelessness'. Taking this concept a practical step further, Calsyn and Morse (1991) have mooted four 'prediction factors' – a lack of human capital, alienation, psychiatric morbidity and stressful life events – as providing a 'diagnosis' of homelessness.

The work in the area of describing homelessness as a medical condition has reached no firm conclusions. This diagnostic 'problem-solving' approach is, however, at the heart of Western medical philosophy. Reducing phenomena to their constituent parts and establishing causal links forms the basis of Cartesian theory and is the classical manner in which disease is addressed (Downie and Telfer 1980, Holmes 1990). Linked to this 'reductionist' approach is the definition of professional responsibility; that is, having diagnosed the condition and its causal links, a professional decision is made regarding the kind of medical intervention that is required and under which speciality the condition should be classified.

The Cartesian process can be straightforward, in the case of a disease caused by a virus for example, where there is a strong causal link between the virus and its effect on the body. It is more difficult when considering conditions that have a societal basis. One example of this is 'baby-battering syndrome', which was recognized in the 1940s not from reports of the actual abuse in the social context but from 'acceptable' physical indicators.

The physical abuse of children was objectively demonstrated when a link was established, in babies admitted to hospital, between subdural haematoma and fractured limbs. This combination of injuries provided tangible, physical evidence that some babies were being systematically physically abused, as it was considered that these injuries could not happen simultaneously by accident (Caffey 1946). This discovery helped to legitimize the professional recognition by the medical profession of the physical abuse of children, even though the abuse of children had been known in the general sense of human experience before that date.

Similarly with homelessness, the medical debate centres around the exact disease patterns of homelessness, their treatment and how the health professions should be involved, that is, what the specific indicators are, which conditions should be treated and which professional or specialist group should take responsibility (Jessop 1987, Connelly et al 1991).

As highlighted earlier, in regard to community care, the precise classification of who is responsible becomes more difficult when there is confusion over whether an individual has a health or a social problem. In these cases, as exemplified in the five projects cited above, health professionals concentrate on those parts of the individual's problems which are specifically health related. In these cases also, the description of the morbidity was very precise – the reduction into constituent parts. However, this process could not be carried through to intervention and cure with the same accuracy as was seen with the other parts of the individual's problem; that is, his or her social context and problems were described in broad imprecise terms. This was seen particularly in the Featherstone and Ashmore (1988) project, in which categories such as 'itinerant' were used alongside precise medical descriptions.

Individuality and expression – Kantian theory

Other literature highlights the difficulties that individuals have in expressing their needs and establishing their rights. These difficulties appear to be complicated by adverse treatment by health professionals (Hudson 1989, Leddington and Shiner 1991). Professional standards and philosophies encourage the approach that all patients should be treated as individuals and equally well (Scottish Home and Health Department 1990), yet it appears that there is a discrepancy between the treatment experiences of different individuals.

Western health service philosophy broadly accepts the Kantian definition of a person as being unique and worthy of individual respect because he or she can (and has a right to) make independent judgements based around self-determination and the formation of ideals. Downie and Telfer (1980) point out that this global belief is tempered in individual cases. The right to individual independence is generally

only bestowed on those who articulate their individuality and, importantly, in the correct manner at the appropriate time and place. People
who cannot or will not articulate their individuality may be treated as a
second- or lower-class persons (Downie and Telfer 1980). Examples
given of these second-class citizens are the mentally handicapped and
the long-term unconscious. They may also be individuals who have
other difficulties in articulation or who are unfamiliar with the form or
etiquette required to achieve a positive outcome. It could be seen in
many of the reports how individuals responded positively to project
workers because they felt more at ease and did not have to engage in,
what were to them, complex negotiations and contractual arrangements to gain mainstream health care (Williams and Allen 1989,
Leddington and Shiner 1991).

Difficulties in expressing need

To articulate one's needs to a statutory service, there are particular
forms of address and behaviour: one must attend the 'appropriate'
agency at the correct time and ask for the service in a prescribed
manner. Second, one's request must be considered relevant and worthy
of attention by the agency. Agencies often have a complex organizational structure, not well understood by those outside. Williams
(1987a), a Plymouth housing officer, describes that whereas rules and
conventions may be obvious and logical within the service, they are
often a complete mystery to those outside, particularly clients.

The appropriateness, or otherwise, of an individual's behaviour
when seeking help from a health service raises questions. If an
individual has a health need, surely he or she is entitled to seek help in
a place dedicated to that purpose? It is difficult to discern from Powell's
(1987a) project how individuals were supposed to know that they were
behaving inappropriately, especially as it may be considered, from the
homeless person's perspective, that A and E has many benefits as it is
open without appointment, one needs to be less articulate and have
fewer negotiating skills, and one receives intervention on the same day.

Utilitarian barriers

The answers to these questions may centre around the individual's
rights being tempered by the perceived rights of the rest of the population – so-called utilitarian philosophy. Citing Locke and J.S. Mill,
Downie and Telfer (1980) and Murdoch (1992) assert that there is a
natural conflict between different individuals and what they and other
people want. Utilitarianism – the striving for the greatest good for the
greatest number of people, coupled with the prerequisite that one

person's right to liberty may not impinge upon another person's similar right to liberty – highlights this conflict. The assumption is that there is a greater good for all and that a level of consensus exists.

The practical effect of these principles is that 'minority' needs may be seen as impinging on the needs of the 'majority'. Their requests may therefore be considered to be 'inappropriate' unless their number becomes great enough to warrant special consideration, as, for example, when the number of homeless families in a London health district increased and policy changes were recommended (Victor et al 1989, Black et al 1991).

Once the individuals are accepted as a discrete group with specific needs large enough for consideration, they are no longer perceived as a minority impinging on the rest. The service may then set standards and practices to cater for the particular group. This may improve the general situation but may work against the individual. For example, Platt (1988) describes how standards to fight against profiteering slum landlords can adversely affect the young single person seeking shelter as it leads to a decrease in the actual number of shelters available.

Respect for the individual's right to 'choose' even an unhealthy lifestyle such as homelessness is also used to justify actions by health professionals (Downie and Telfer 1980). An assumption may be made by the professional that the individual does not want help. He or she has made the same sort of choice with the same range of options as the professional makes when buying a house or choosing a healthy lifestyle for example. This outlook may be compounded by another assumption – that some patients are intrinsically 'worthwhile'. A successful professional may be perceived as 'going somewhere' and being more worthy, while the homeless man is not considered 'worthwhile' (Beauchamp and Perlin 1978, Boss 1979).

Nursing and moral knowledge

Interventions or projects described in the literature were considered to be successful if they produced a positive or curative outcome, that is, if a resolution was achieved (Powell 1987a, 1987b, Williams and Allen 1989); in the project evaluations, just 'being with' the homeless people was not in itself seen as a measure of success. On a practical level, the measurement of interactions assists one in gauging a project's efficacy and relevance to practice. It also helps to establish a profession's 'right' to operate. The medical profession, in order to justify its existence, generally has to 'prove' that there is disease present, with causal relationships between pathology and cure (Holmes 1990).

Justifying nursing intervention has been shown to have a different emphasis. 'Curing' is an important basis for nursing intervention (Greene 1979), but there are also others. Carper (1978) agrees that nursing action derives from empirical knowledge, that is, research-based knowledge that includes the knowledge of causal and curative relationships in order to guide interventions. Carper (1978) also states that nursing practice derives from three other sources of knowledge: aesthetic knowledge, which is associated with human creativity and which recognizes the art or craft of nursing practice; personal knowledge, which is demonstrated in the unique contribution that an individual makes to nursing practice; and moral knowledge, which forms the basis of acting because something is considered 'right', that is, from an ethical basis.

Bearing witness

The above four knowledge bases have relevance in the justification of nursing practice. Other nursing literature recognizes moral knowledge as a part of practice (Sarvimaki 1988). A nurse may sometimes act because she thinks that the action is ethical rather than primarily because the intervention will be curative. At a primary level, the nurse may attend the patient simply acting upon a moral conviction that she should be wherever the patients are. To become involved with an individual or group, a nurse may not have to justify her actions by immediately demonstrating effective curative practice, although efficacy is beneficial to the patient and to the service. Certainly, when the author first started his work with homeless men, he could not have asserted that he was being either effective or curative. He did, however, act from a strong motivation that he should be present with these men, to witness and describe what he saw.

Practice patterns of shared time

The concept of 'being there' is supported by patterns of time spent with the patient by nurses and doctors. Bishop and Scudder (1990) describe how a doctor's time with the patient tends to be intermittent, dictated by the agenda of treating the disease, usually via appointments. He or she will seldom speak with or be in the presence of the patient unless it is for a specific purpose. This highly focused approach tends to limit the interaction between the two as people.

A nurse may spend more continuous time with the patient because he or she is often in the patient's physical company while attending to other duties involving either the patient or another person. A shared experience of the physical and human environment may enable different relationships and a deeper knowledge of each other to ensue, and may enable the nurse to enter more fully into the patient's experience. This deeper knowledge of the complexities of a person's life and health experience can also include an acceptance that 'progress' may not be possible, that the patient's life is painful and has irresolvable problems (Barker 1989). A formal recognition of the effects of spiritual concepts such as hope is also possible in this multidimensional framework (Stephenson 1991). By witnessing the patient's life on this basis, nurses may be able to represent the individual's needs with accuracy and insight (Davis 1986).

Summary

For the purposes of the study, this brief philosophical examination was deemed to be useful as it helped to provide direction and purpose for the study. The study would describe the individual residents' situation in as holistic a way as possible within a social context, representing, whenever possible, the complex and conflicting experiences they faced. This would not be possible if the study sought and described only morbidity by screening and reporting the outcomes of interventions.

Theoretical framework of the study

Function of the theoretical framework

As the literature review and preparatory work progressed, it became apparent that two quite different perspectives could be taken in the study. First (and particularly highlighted in the literature from Shelter and the voluntary agencies) were the stories of individuals, how homelessness affected them and how they responded to their situation and sought help. Second (particularly in the clinical and professional literature) there were the descriptions of homeless people as groups, attitudes towards these groups and how these groups behaved, appropriately or otherwise, towards the main community.

The five projects cited above highlighted health professionals interacting with homeless people, but whereas the clinical descriptions were informative, there was little description (with the exception of Williams and Allen 1989) of the actual individuals and their experience, either personally or as a group. Williams and Allen (1989) used individuals' comments and statements to highlight key areas, but they did not form part of the analysis, nor did they give any insight into how these individuals lived or any rationale for their actions.

It was thus considered important to bring into the study theoretical perspectives that would assist in analysing the data and presenting a more complete picture of the men individually and severally, interacting between themselves, as well as of their environment and the health professionals who attempted to help them. This section, therefore, highlights the interface between the individual and his social context – the men as a group – along with the effects of illness on both his and the group's actions. The juxtaposition of the individual and the group forms the basis for the study's theoretical framework.

The theoretical framework is based on the nursing theory of Roy (1980) and the sociological study of the group, which includes aspects of deviancy theory. It must be emphasized that the main source of knowledge in this study was to be gained by the empirical work, going out into the field, collecting data and analysing this evidence.

The theoretical framework, as with the philosophical examination, provides an important supporting role in gaining insight into the data. The study does not, therefore, set out to assert or disavow the theories, but to use them as 'lenses' through which to examine the data from different perspectives.

Having stated the purpose of the theoretical framework, this section and the analysis in Chapters 8 and 9 will highlight areas of tension where the literature or the data appear to contrast with the theory. It is hoped that this will provide a further insight into the lives of the men in the study sample.

The first of these areas of tension is that Roy's (1980) theory and the school of thought known as deviancy theory are not primarily based on the specific observation of study samples. They are instead based on an intellectual interpretation of physical and societal phenomena examined and presented in a universal manner; that is, they refer to humanity in general, although specific examples are cited. Roy (in Roy and Andrews 1991) describes how she used the observation of 500 patients to categorize her 'adaptive modes', but her theory was formed as a result of theological and philosophical study and reflection.

Such theories have led to movements or 'schools' of thought that have taken the original concepts to further levels and diversions, particularly in deviancy theory. This study has not engaged in the process of taking the theories to new levels but has concentrated on using the theories to improve knowledge about the sample group. To achieve this, the study has, therefore, aimed to adhere to the original or basic principles of the theories rather than later interpretations and critiques.

Introduction to the study's theoretical framework

Apparently paradoxical behaviour of individuals regarding their health

An apparent paradox may sometimes be seen when an individual becomes ill and reacts to the illness, or when he is confronted by strategies to promote a healthy lifestyle. Whetstone and Reid (1991) observe that if one places a high priority on good health, one should, in theory, maintain a healthy life style. This is patently not the case as people engage in physically and mentally damaging behaviour even if they state that health is a priority.

Merely being told or having knowledge that one is ill and being told what to do does not appear sufficient. There appears to be a barrier between an individual's having knowledge and his or her transfer of that knowledge into action. People also appear to make negative, or self-harming, adaptations regarding their own health and lifestyle. Perceiving this behaviour as paradoxical may be seen as a result of using a reductionist model to analyse an individual's response to knowledge. In a seminal paper, Phillips (1977, p 356) explains it thus:

> The medical model posits a dichotomy between mind and body which is not congruent with the philosophy of nursing in its concern for the whole person. Not only is nursing concerned with the structure and function of the body but also with human experience, behaviour, feelings, and the influence of social forces upon the body – manifestations of the man–environment interaction, whether they be termed normal or abnormal.

In this quotation, the 'structure and function of the body' may be seen to represent the search for morbidity, the 'human experience, behaviour, feelings' to represent the individual's response, and the 'influence of social forces upon the body' the group and society's effect on the individual and each other.

Taking these factors together, the simplistic paradox cited earlier is placed into a more intricate context. Resolution is not just a matter of knowledge + action = cure; the factors are interlinked. Nursing theoretical models strive to represent the interaction of these factors while presenting the systematic means to put them into action.

It should be emphasized that although the quotation above encapsulates the drive for holism in nursing practice and theory, it may be criticized for polarizing medical and nursing practice as if medical practice is entirely reductionist and nursing entirely holistic. More recent literature demonstrates that both professions use these elements in a more integrated way. Stern and Stillwell (1989) in particular demonstrate how medical and nursing practitioners, as equal partners, may work together in delivering health care for homeless people. The quotation does, however, demonstrate the principles of holistic care on which nursing theories are based.

Background to nursing models

Representing the complexity of the interaction of the individual's body and mind with his social and environmental context has led to the development of certain nursing 'models' that are based on theories from different academic perspectives (Ingram 1991, Reed and Robbins 1991). The individual may be viewed through his daily activities (Roper et al 1990) or as normally functional and self-caring (Orem 1995). Another model perceives the human being as an integrated physiological musculoskeletal structure (Akinsanya 1987). Roy (1980) regards the person as a social being interacting with physical and social phenomena.

The brief descriptions in this paragraph may make the differences between these approaches stark, but there is a measure of consensus in all models in that their purpose is to guide the practitioner by encouraging a multiperspective analysis of the patient (Fawcett 1992).

Roy's adaptation theory and model

For this study, Roy's nursing theory of adaptation has been chosen as it considers the individual as an adaptive physical and psychosocial being (Roy 1980, Johnson 1991). The individual is considered in four 'adaptive modes'(Roy 1980, Aggleton and Chalmers 1986):

1. physiological, pertaining to function, anatomy and illness;
2. self-concept, that is, an individual's opinion of himself and his experience of social engagement and disengagement;
3. role function, which is how the individual behaves and adapts as a member of society with duties and responsibilities, for example as a father or family member;
4. interdependency, which describes the individual as an integrated community member and any dysfunction he may experience, such as rejection by others.

Scientific and philosophical assumptions

These four adaptive modes are underpinned by scientific and philo-sophical assumptions. The individual is a biopsychosocial being inter-acting with his changing environment all the time, using acquired and innate strategies derived from these three parts of his being. One inevitable dimension to his existence is health and illness. To respond positively to this and his environment, it is necessary for the person to adapt. Adaptations are a function and product of stimuli experienced, which exert tensions and stresses, and the person's adaptation level, which registers the range of stimulation and degree of stress that is likely to produce a positive response (Roy 1980).

Humanist principles

In philosophical terms, the theory and model are based on four humanist principles and four truths, which Roy calls principles of 'veritivity'. It should be stated here that the philosophical assumptions have only been expressed precisely over recent years as a result of the theory's wide dissemination and subsequent debate (Roy 1988).

In summary, the humanist principles recognize that a person behaves purposefully (rather than empirically following a line of causes and effects), that he possesses 'intrinsic holism' and that he is driven to keep his integrity in a context of meaningful relationships with other people. Roy also states that the individual shares with others in the power to create.

Veritivity

The four truths are connected to the humanist principles. In turn, they are based on Roy's basic assumption that absolute truth exists (veritivity) and that human existence shares a 'common purposeful-ness'. An individual may therefore be considered within these four terms of reference, which highlight the purposefulness of existence, the unity of man's purpose, his activity and creativity for life, and the common good containing value and meaning.

Relevance of Roy's theory

Roy's (1980) theory is relevant in relation to the single homeless men in this study. As has been described in the five projects cited above, homeless individuals were found with a variety of physical and psychi-atric illnesses. They lived in 'bad' conditions, yet there seemed little evidence of responding to these obvious stimuli. The questions raised here centre around whether it was a case of the service not responding to the men or whether the men were making few or indeed different responses to these stimuli. This study examines the responses of the men to their circumstances and evidence of purposeful activity seeking companionship and interacting with other people.

Also relevant to this study is the consideration of the individual as a higher being rather than merely a functional or dysfunctional organism in need of 'mending'. Concepts such as common purpose and absolute truth, which may be laudable, appeared to need examination and challenge in the context of caring for homeless people as their accounts, and the experience of the authors of the project reports, portrayed a grim picture in many cases. The use of Roy's (1980) theory as an analytical device to examine the data was of help in examining the individuals' experience in relation to these 'higher' concepts, which could bring further insight into the men's individual humanity.

A sociological perspective on the study of the group

The literature has demonstrated some aspects of homelessness, particularly in relation to single homeless men. A high incidence of psychiatric and physical morbidity was discovered in the five clinical projects examined in this thesis and in other reports. It has also been demonstrated that health services should, in theory and by law, be available to these men, yet it is apparent that these services have difficulty delivering care despite some examples of positive innovatory work.

Roy's (1980) theory and model concentrates on the individual's adaptation to physiological, environmental and psychological stimuli. There is a body of knowledge that considers group responses to social and disease forces. In hospitals, especially long-stay hospitals for example, institutionalization, dependency and depersonalization have been recognized and observed in long-stay patients, but there appear to be parallels for hostel-dwelling men, particularly the loss of their individual independence and their behaviour being interpreted as group behaviour. This behaviour is often perceived by health and other services to be 'inappropriate' (Smith 1981).

Deviancy theory

Deviancy theory has been described as a misnomer as it is not a single perspective but a combination of conflicting views concentrating on sociological criminology and the concept of rule-breaking (Downes and Rock 1982). Because of the diversity of views, it is important to express the specific relevance of deviancy to this study.

Deviancy theory considers groups who behave in an aberrant or deviant manner towards the society in which they live, as well as factors such as the functional role of institutions (for example, hospitals and hostels) in maintaining a well-ordered society. The theory centres around the concept that groups and societies have a number of values and norms of behaviour to which they adhere. Certain individuals break these rules either by their actions or by their lifestyles. These people may be seen as deviants (Redhead 1984).

Some of the observations made in the evaluation reports cited in this chapter group the men as 'itinerant', 'disorganized' and 'alcoholic' (Featherstone and Ashmore 1988) alongside their specific clinical findings. This classification and labelling by the main community of smaller groups in this way is a key feature of deviancy theory. Although in recent years it has become less fashionable in sociological and health circles, labelling is still current in everyday practice and is recognized in recent studies as an essential feature in progress and outcome for these groups. Jenkins (1996) describes how the labels may be authoritatively imposed onto those in an institutional setting and outlines the tension created by the difference between the definition that one gives oneself and that given by others. Aronson (1991), in his examination of deviance, observes that individuals and groups are motivated by the desire to correct or change for the better (usually in private behaviour) and the desire to remain in the good graces of others (usually manifested in public behaviour)

These elements of sociological and deviancy theory posed interesting questions for the study. Were the men itinerant? Did they define themselves as a group? Did they have similar perceptions of themselves in relationship to their environment and the main community? Did they consider themselves as homeless? Did they choose their circumstances and the group, or was this period of their life an aberration? Bordieu (1990) describes 'habitus' – the domain of habit, which is created both individually and collectively; was the men's lifestyle merely dictated by habit and a collective sharing of their own or a rejection of others' values?

The relevance of these and other questions and their answers could provide an insight into the motivations of the men, their underlying needs (as opposed to just their presenting symptoms) and possible ways of adapting practice to coincide with their requirements. A sociological theoretical perspective was used both in the formation of the study questionnaire and in the analysis of the data (described in Chapter 9).

Joint objectives of Roy's theory and deviancy theory

Deviancy also considers groups of people in conflict or co-operation with one another. Some groups are seen to deviate from 'normal' behaviour in response to the dominant group. The group may reject society by its behaviour and by eschewing help.

Roy's (1980) and deviancy theory each enable an examination both of the barriers that may exist for the men in obtaining health services and of the barriers that services place before the men. These barriers may be termed 'internal', emanating from the individual and his perception, or 'external', coming from professionals within the services, who may prevent access or make it difficult to obtain.

Conflict between the individual and the services is described in several areas of study. Roth (1963) describes the interaction between doctor and patient. He describes how 'making deals' occurs as the doctor, addressing the needs of the disease, bargains with the patient who has his own agenda (Roth 1963).

Relevance of comparison with other marginalized groups

It is important to place the examination of the residents in this study against the wider context of other groups. Simply probing into the sample's experience would make it difficult to highlight the relevance of the men's position, particularly in relation to service delivery. Central to this section of the study of the literature was to discover whether their experience was unique and whether insights from this and the experience of other studies might be focused on practical outcomes for marginalized groups, including the homeless.

The literature demonstrates a pattern of circumstances and experience in different groups of people who may be termed deviant and who are subsequently 'marginalized'. In a radio talk in 1991, the Anglican Archbishop of Durham, David Jenkins, termed these individuals 'those who have been pushed out, left out or who have dropped out'.

Certainly, from a health professional standpoint, there appear to be similarities between the health and service experience of people such as ethnic minorities (O'Meachair and Burns 1988, Black Housing 1989), travelling people (Rickford and Montague 1987, Streetly 1987), prisoners (Brimacombe 1990), the mentally ill and handicapped (Rappaport 1981, Morfett and Pidgeon 1991), the disabled (Barnes 1991) and the 'poor' (Kitching 1991).

Connections between the homeless and other institutions

Literature emanating from practitioners and organizations in the homeless and community care fields show connections between homeless men, prisoners, mental illness and institutions (Brimacombe 1990, McMillan 1991). This appears to be borne out by the literature examining morbidity, particularly mental illness and deviancy (Gove 1982). Historical evidence is also cited demonstrating changing societal attitudes towards alcohol abuse, for example, and its concomitant effects on lifestyle (Conrad and Schneider 1980).

The reported attitudes of service professionals appear to have resonances with one aspect of deviancy – control theory – which advocates the regulation of institutions as the cornerstone of a well-ordered society. Functionalism, conversely, may view the hostel-dwellers' lifestyle as a necessary 'evil', providing an important, if negative, function and role in society (Downes and Rock 1982). Health assumptions and philosophies, in this context, aim to intervene and interact to restore functionality. Recent studies have also made a connection between deviance and social bonds made in adult life, such as in employment and in the family (Robins Lee and Rutter 1990, Sampson and Laub 1990). Aspects of this connection will be exemplified in Chapter 9.

Individuals belonging to several marginalized groups

Relevant to this study is the effect on an individual of being homeless and belonging to one or more other marginalized groups. O'Meachair and Burns (1988) describe the particular difficulties of Irish men in London and their overrepresentation among the single homeless. Barnes (1991) describes the problems that the disabled have with housing and homelessness because of discrimination and low employment possibilities.

The National Council for Voluntary Organisations (1988) reflects that statutory provision for the disadvantaged, including the homeless, needs special consideration. Central policy-makers have difficulty developing strategy for these groups. This may be because of an incomplete knowledge of their needs. It also appears that because certain individuals have been placed in 'groups' by others, there is an assumption that the groups are homogeneous. Policy may then be based on stereotypical views rather than a response to individuals (Black Housing 1989, Barnes 1991).

Many of the problems described as relating to homeless people are common to others; these are exemplified below. Some of the factors bear closer examination, which broadens the relevance of the project and extends the areas in which information has been gained.

Unemployment and poverty

Homeless people are found to have limited access to employment and are often disadvantaged by sickness, disability and old age (Sanders 1990, Whynes 1990). Oppenheim (1991), writing on behalf of the organization the Child Poverty Action Group, uses exactly these criteria to describe the principle causes of poverty.

Family breakdown

Other factors include domestic disruption and the loss of family or social context. The high number of homeless people whose situation has been caused or influenced by family breakdown or the loss of a significant partner exemplifies this point (Shelter 1988). Atkinson and Thompson (1989) also describe elderly people on their caseloads who, while still living in their own houses, have lost their families, neighbours, local amenities, health and mobility. These individuals demonstrate many of the problems of the poor and homeless.

Ostracized individuals

The ostracism of homeless individuals by mainstream services, as well as families and individuals, has been described (Laing 1993). Another example is of the Home Office, who recognized how mentally ill black people often receive adverse treatment and are commonly treated as criminals. In Circular 66/90, the courts were directed to divert the mentally ill from prisons (Medical Campaign Project and Campaign for Homeless and Rootless 1991). Common throughout the literature is reference to inappropriate responses to individual needs and a lack of resources, in conjunction with a lack of articulation skills in the marginalized, and compounded by a perception that there is a lack of political will to do anything about the problems (Julty 1981, Edwards 1986).

Regulations: their effect on the marginalized

Perhaps the most significant area of commonality between marginalized people is the effect of statutory regulation and provision. For example, providing an individual has a registered address (which can be a hostel), he or she should be able to register on a GP's caseload. This having been achieved, the individual is, in theory and by law, entitled to the same primary health care as any other member of the population (Bayliss and Logan 1987, Stern 1990), yet marginalized people have difficulty in acquiring services and legal recognition that should be theirs by right. Others appear not to receive timeous, adequate standards of service delivery, which, had they been members of the general population, they would have received promptly (Baine and Benington 1992).

A dramatic example of this is Standard Minimum Rules for the Treatment of Prisoners. At the first United Nations (UN) Congress on the Prevention of Crime and the Treatment of Offenders in 1955,

Article 9 states that 'each prisoner shall occupy by night a cell or room by himself' (CIBA Foundation 1973, pp 199–200). Article 12 states that prisoners should be able to comply with the needs of nature 'when necessary and in a clean and decent manner'. These resolutions were adopted by the UN on 30 August 1955. It is interesting to observe that in 2000, prisoners in Britain were still sleeping two or more to a cell and were still 'slopping out'. Similar below-standard conditions prevail in much homeless accommodation despite health and safety legislation (Atkinson 1987, Donaghue 1989, Houghton and Timperley 1992).

Falling outside the regulations

Even when laws are passed catering for specific groups, problems still arise. The Joint Charities Group on Homelessness reported that the 1985 Housing Act, Part III of which replaced the 1977 (Homeless Persons) Act, had six main 'drawbacks'. These included the fact that many homeless people, particularly single homeless, were not incorporated in the Act. Other literature describes how new groups of marginalized and homeless are created by new legislation, specifically the removal of benefits for youths of 16–18 years of age (Smith 1989, Nelson and Kirk 1991) and inadequate community care for the mentally ill (Weller and Weller 1988).

Appropriate use of services: different agendas

Different agendas are reflected in health service research studies in which those providing the services decide what is 'appropriate' use and then conduct research with groups, such as the homeless, who are considered to be acting inappropriately (Powell 1987a, Black et al 1991). The literature did not appear to address these issues in a systematic way. Service-based studies tended to examine provision and uptake, as well as the physical and practical barriers to achieving this.

The 'appropriate' use of services is coupled with correct diagnosis: individuals seeking help may be told that they are not ill, for example. Foucault (1973, p95) describes how disease comprises not only its manifest symptoms, but also its description; that is, it must be seen and spoken. In order to arrive at a correct diagnosis, the individual with the disease must be able to describe in the correct terms what his problem is (overcoming internal barriers). This is as important as it is for the doctor to be able to observe and recognize the symptoms. By using Roy's theory, insight may be gained regarding the internal barriers, with a focus on the individual. Deviancy theory provides an insight into the homeless men as a group interacting with the service delivery group. An examination of these interactions will take place in Chapter 9.

Summary and conclusion

This chapter has, by reviewing the literature, attempted to provide a foundation for the study and place it in the context of related work by other health professionals with a conceptual framework within which to proceed with the study. Homelessness has been described in general terms and with reference to the more specific areas of single homeless men and the situation in Glasgow. The purpose of the literature review was to inform the design of the study by seeking out the areas that research and other publications had highlighted as requiring further examination:

- that because there are many definitions of 'homeless', the terms of reference for this study would refer to a group of single homeless men living in homeless accommodation, namely a hostel;
- that further, detailed work with individual homeless people was needed;
- that the study should follow a group of individuals through a process of assessment, intervention and evaluation;
- that the relationship between homelessness and health, with its concomitant effects on single homeless men, should if possible be described;
- that the philosophical and theoretical analysis demonstrated the possibility of studying the men both as individuals (using Roy's theory), gaining an insight into their perceptions, and as a group interacting with their social context (using a sociological analysis including deviancy theory);
- that the study should contain a systematic evaluation of district nursing intervention with individuals in this group;
- that gaining access to mainstream health services by any member of the population requires that they have a registered address and a GP. It was found that most single homeless men in Glasgow met these criteria, yet men were found to have difficulty gaining access to health services. There also appeared to be resistance from some men to go to their doctor to receive care. Insight into the reasons for these anomalies was necessary.

This study therefore attempts to address these important areas in a systematic manner, using both a quantitative and a qualitative research design.

Chapter 3

Research design, method and pilot study

This book reports on a descriptive and evaluative study of district nursing intervention with single homeless men that utilized both quantitative and qualitative methods. To this end, the first section of this chapter describes the research design, method and preparation of the study, the second the fieldwork.

Two nurses were involved in the fieldwork: the author of the study, who undertook the interviews in the Comparison Hostel and also interviewed the doctors and nurses, and the project nurse, who was employed by the study to undertake the assessments and interventions in the Main Study Hostel. A full description of the rationale behind the roles of the two nurses is given at the end of the first section.

Design, method and preparation

This section will present the study design, methods and preparation in the following order:

- Aims and objectives
- Methods:
    - Profile of the Main Study Hostel and Comparison Hostel
    - Data-gathering of the residents' demographic characteristics
    - Assessment of the residents – assumptions
    - Possibility of intervention
    - Intervention
    - Evaluation
- Separation of assessment and intervention from evaluation
- Ethical principles.

As will be seen, this study comprises many interlinking parts. To clarify its design, Figure 3.1 provides a diagrammatic summary.

Main Study Hostel: administered by project nurse, structured interview		Comparison Hostel: administered by author, structured interview	
Part One Demographic questionnaire *Part Two* Validated tools		*Part One* Questionnaire *Part Two* Validated tools	
Main study proceeds to assessment		**Comparison study ceases**	
Assessment: administered by project nurse structured interview *Part Three* Mental status questionnaire (over 60s) Semi-structured interview **Nursing assessment** If resident does not require intervention: **Interview Ceases** If resident does require intervention, study proceeds to **intervention**			
Intervention: administered by project nurse *Part Four* Planning intervention **Intervention**			
Evaluation: administered by author Semi-structured interviews with health workers *Part Five* Evaluation			
Expert panel: facilitated by project nurse Written and taped responses of six district nurses presented with six anonymized case histories			

Figure 3.1: Diagrammatic summary of the study

Aims and objectives

Aims

From the study of the literature and the preparatory work, the formal aims of the study were developed.

1. To record the health status of the men in the Main Study Hostel and of men in a comparison group.
2. To record the health-related difficulties experienced by the men in the Main Study Hostel and to make interventions.
3. To evaluate the effect of district nursing interventions with the men in the Main Study Hostel.

4. To develop new nursing and related knowledge and to make recommendations.

Objectives

To achieve the aims, the following objectives were set:

1. To describe the demographic details of the men in the Main Study Hostel and to compare these with the demographic profiles of men in the Comparison Hostel.
2. To undertake nursing assessments of the residents in the Main Study Hostel.
3. Where necessary, to implement interventions (treatments, referrals and acts of advocacy) following the nursing assessment.
4. To evaluate referrals by interviewing the relevant doctors and nurses.

The study aimed to discover physical and psychiatric morbidity in two ways: first, through the individual residents expressing problems to the nurse, and second, through the nurse's discovering hidden or unexpressed morbidity during the nursing assessment interview and by the use of validated tools.

It was decided that although the discovery of morbidity was important, it should, as far as possible, always be within the context of the individual man's expressed need and understanding. This was in line with the findings of other projects, cited in Chapter 2, in which better outcomes were seen when patients understood the effects of any intervention. Thus, for example, it was decided in this study not to use invasive procedures, i.e. not to take blood or urine samples or measure other vital signs.

Methods

Profile of the Main Study Hostel and Comparison Hostel

Exploratory work, negotiation of access and information

To begin the study, it was important to explore the possibility of undertaking the research, in a rigorous manner, within the restrictions of this difficult area of practice. Nothing could be taken for granted. Access at all levels had to be negotiated and was always time-consuming. Every aspect of the study had to be tested in terms of its feasibility and the reliability of the data gained.

By interviewing hostel managers and other workers in the field, and from the author's previous experience, it was decided to gather the information about the men in the largest commercial hostel in

Glasgow (referred to as the Main Study Hostel) over a period of approximately 12 weeks. This would provide a 'snapshot' of a particular group of men so that they would be, as far as possible, the same group of men throughout the study.

Negotiations to gain access and co-operation were undertaken in the Main Study Hostel. The hostel is famous throughout Scotland and is also very busy. It has been running for a number of years and has an open admission policy; that is, unless an individual has been barred for bad behaviour, a man can register for a bed from the street. Some of the council-run hostels have an admission system via other admission hostels. Access and permission to practise as a district nurse was received from the hostel management. Contacts were made with Social Services Homeless Unit, the GCSH and the GDC Hostels Unit. These agencies all employ dedicated personnel working with homeless men. The purpose of this activity was to facilitate access to the group and to gain more detailed information about the difficulties the men experienced.

Comparison group

As the study design developed, and taking into account the desire to demonstrate the study's relevance to other health professionals and groups, it was considered vital to compare the main sample with another. It was not possible to form a representative sample or a control group as one could not guarantee that individuals selected for the potential sample groups would take part; also very little information was available about individual residents, particularly in the Main Study Hostel. The study did, however, gain access to another, similarly sized hostel, which was run by the GDC (referred to as the Comparison Hostel). The study attempted to recruit a similar number of men in this hostel as a comparison sample.

Further preparatory work in the hostels and with Glasgow agencies

Apart from the review of the literature and the development of the academic format of the study, there was a great deal of practical organization and refinement to be undertaken. This was made more important for the following reasons.

First, while it was part of some community nurses' practice to go into hostels, it was not a large part of their remit. As with any other residence or home, they had no automatic right of admission, having to have an invitation from the individual resident and/or the permission of the hostel management. This was made more apparent as the Main Study Hostel was privately owned. Thus, the proposed method of working, which involved a regular district nursing presence in the hostel, was an entirely new approach for both the residents and the management. The author had to negotiate to ensure that this changed role for district nurses was acceptable to all involved with the hostel.

Second, the policy of the hostels and GDC Hostels Unit was to ensure complete confidentiality for all residents. Accordingly, there was no exchange of information about individual residents, as is the custom between many health agencies. This is not a criticism but demonstrates that the study worked from an 'outsider's' position. Access to important information for the study therefore had to be negotiated and had to depend upon methods other than formal records.

Third, the author, an experienced district nurse, was used to working in a team and accustomed to being welcomed in health service settings and given access. However, in the 'outsider' position, no assumptions about automatic access could be made, and respect and trust had to be earned. This took time and patience over a number of visits.

There had previously been various surveys of the Main Study Hostel (Glasgow Council for Single Homeless 1991). These had not, however, involved the amount of interaction with residents that was necessary for this study. The author thus had to spend a great deal of time in different hostels observing, listening, talking and working out possibilities for the study's pattern of practice.

Sources of information

As has been mentioned, it was found in the initial investigation that very little was known about each man in the Main Study Hostel, although age, length of stay and GP were known in relation to all the residents. Unfortunately, this information was not known for all residents in the Comparison Hostel. There was, therefore, no central source of information about individuals so information would have to be gleaned by the study from each individual. A wide-ranging, but concise, questionnaire would thus be necessary to address the aims and specific objectives within the time parameters.

Contemporaneous record of visits to hostels by other health professionals

During the study, a record was kept of any visits made to the hostel by other professionals that had not been directly influenced by the study. This information was obtained from the hostel staff, its purpose being to ascertain an impression of the usual activity of health professionals in the hostels.

Data-gathering of the residents' demographic characteristics

Demographic description

In order to determine whether the residents in the study location were typical of the homeless population as a whole, it was important to place the work and the Main Study Hostel within the context of the homeless scene in general and Glasgow in particular. The contacts made with the various statutory and voluntary agencies made it possible to gain access to information regarding all the homeless hostels in Glasgow, the number of men, turnover, living conditions, conditions of entry, services available and staffing level. With these data, it was possible to compare the residents of the Main Study Hostel with others in similar circumstances. This process ensured that the generalizability of the research results could be assessed in the future.

Sample

It was not possible to select a reliable cross-section of the hostel residents as it was not known what attrition rate there would be. It was thus decided to attempt to interview as many men as possible (170 men being the usual number in residence) at the Main Study Hostel in the 12-week period of the fieldwork rather than set an arbitrary sample size. Information would be gained about each resident so that an accurate profile of the hostel and its residents would emerge. Each resident would be asked to join the study.

Comparison sample

The study aimed to examine one establishment in detail and place the men in the context of age, family status, employment and other demographic factors. These factors would be tested for typicality by comparing them with another group of hostel residents from the Comparison Hostel, who would be interviewed but would not receive nursing assessments or interventions.

It was recognized by the author, as well as by his academic and funding supervisors, that the two groups who agreed to participate were not necessarily representative of the total population in the two hostels or that one group was a control. There was also no attempt to set up matched pairs of residents (their details being confidential and access limited). Establishing this would therefore have been unwieldy and impracticable.

The results of the study will thus be carefully interpreted in the light of a possible bias. In order to identify the nature of this possible bias, information on age for those who did not take part was obtained. It should, however, be acknowledged that those men who did not take part may have had significant health-related problems undiscovered by the study.

It was also decided that, in practical terms, there would be a better response if all the residents were approached and invited to take part, although it was expected that a large number would not want to take part. Other projects had had similar logistical experiences (Powell 1987b, Williams and Allen 1989).

These logistic considerations indicated that approximately 14 men per week would have to be recruited to the study and approximately three per day interviewed. Taking into account the fact that the recruiting would take time, it was considered that the interviews, particularly those which did not result in assessment for intervention, should take half an hour, but it was decided that an upper limit of 1 hour per person was acceptable.

The questionnaire

The questionnaire (see Appendix I) was developed by the author over many months from the examination of the literature and by addressing the need to discover personal information about the individual residents and their lives, as well as to provide a profile of the men as a group. The questionnaire was to be administered by the author and project nurse in order to assist men who had reading difficulties and to aid clarity. The answers would then form the main database of the study. Many questions were written, of which 26 were finally chosen. Each question had to:

- be easily understood by the subjects with the minimum of explanation;
- have specific relevance to the individual and form the first part of the nursing assessment;
- enable frequency calculations and comparisons, for example regarding age, the length of stay in hostels, the last time treatment was received or distance from GP.

In addition, the 26 main questions (the variables) and the possible categories of answer (the values) had to be mutually exclusive, unequivocal and able to be expressed as a number on a data spreadsheet (Statistical Package for the Social Sciences 1990).

It is important to emphasize at this stage that the answers to the questionnaire and the scores of the validated tools performed two functions: first, to act as the first part of an individual nursing assessment, and second, to provide statistical data for comparative analysis.

Bearing this in mind, and within the constraints of the time available for each interview, great effort went into the selection of the validated tools. The questionnaire and validated tools were piloted to test their ease of use and relevance in the field (see above).

Barthel Index

One of the main difficulties to be overcome was the validity of any information gathered regarding function. Most validated quality of life and function measures depend on some assumptions of social context. Some assessment tools in common use within the health services were found to be inappropriate when considering single homeless men living on their own. For example, one section of the popular and effective Nottingham Quality of Life Profile asks whether the person's health affects his work, holidays and relationships with others. A negative answer from hostel residents was more likely to indicate a lack of relevance to their lifestyle rather than being of significance for their state of health (Hunt 1981).

It was decided, therefore, to use the Barthel Index (see Appendix I), which is a simple scoring system that concentrates only on physical function (Mahoney and Barthel 1965). This well-validated tool has been used in hospitals and, of particular relevance to this study, in community settings (McAndrew and Hanley 1988). It examines mobility, continence and the ability to wash and dress, providing a score ranging from zero to 100 in which 100 denotes full physical function and zero no physical function. The score was incorporated into the statistical analysis.

Hospital Anxiety and Depression scale

Similarly, psychiatric morbidity has been shown in the literature to be an important feature of the experience of homeless people (Hamid and McCarthy 1989, Williams and Allen 1989). Again, it was important to provide a description of which residents were affected by psychiatric illness and anxiety as opposed to 'normal' dissatisfaction with their present circumstances. One well-validated tool is the Hospital Anxiety and Depression (HAD) scale (Zigmond and Snaith 1983).

The main feature of this tool is that it isolates feelings of anxiety from those of biogenic depression. This was an important feature for the study, as the scale identifies those who are suffering from anhedonia (a loss of the ability to experience pleasure), which is indicative of biogenic depression and distinguishes those who may be reactively depressed (as a result of their environment, for example). People who are biogenically depressed are recognized as being good candidates for medication and psychiatric treatment; that is, they are likely to experience a positive outcome from these interventions (Zigmond and Snaith 1983, Snaith 1991).

The HAD scale has been used in many hospital and community settings, particularly in outpatient departments, not dissimilar to the interview situation of the project nurse and author (Goldberg 1985). It comprises 14 straightforward, that is not medically expressed, questions, and provides two scores, one for anxiety and the other for depression. These scores, ranging from zero to 21, zero being low and 21 high in relation to levels of anxiety and depression, were also incorporated into the statistical package and analysis (see Appendix I).

Impact of Alcohol on Lifestyle Questionnaire and Amount of Smoking Questionnaire

Both in popular assumption and in the literature, reference has been made to the connection between homeless men and alcohol (British Broadcasting Corporation 1987, Powell 1987a). Many of the men whom the author had met had previously suffered from alcohol-related problems. It was decided to quantify this factor as far as possible by finding out not simply how much alcohol each resident consumed, but also its effect on lifestyle and experience.

A questionnaire was developed from Skinner's Drug and Alcohol (MAST and DAST) Questionnaires (the language being changed slightly to ensure clarity for the sample), which highlight the effects of substance use rather than the amount consumed (Skinner 1982). The questions examined the effects of alcohol use on relationships, events involving the law, prison and hospital, patterns of alcohol intake, and amount of alcohol intake in units. The variety of questions, with their cumulative scores, was intended to paint a realistic picture of the individual resident's experience and the probable effects of alcohol intake. One event, by itself, would not 'label' an individual.

The first part of the study was common to the samples in the Main Study Hostel and the Comparison Hostel. The rest of the study, that is, the nursing assessment and intervention, took place with the sample from the Main Study Hostel only.

Nursing assessment of the residents

Assumptions

In order to achieve the study objectives, it would be necessary for each man to receive an extensive assessment (see Appendix I). These assessments were based on the recognition that health status and quality of life are linked, and that factors such as an individual's mental function and his interaction with his physical and social environment are as important as the recording of physical clinical signs (Andrews and Withey 1976, Granger and Greer 1976, Hunt and McEwen 1980, Sintonen 1981, Heptinstall 1989, Hughes 1992). Implicit is the assumption that the individual's subjective view of his status has the same relevance to his assessment as does an objective diagnosis by a health professional (George 1981, McKenna et al 1981, Diener 1984, Royal College of Physicians and British Geriatrics Society 1992).

Assessment process

As stated above, the questionnaire and validated tools also provided the first part of a nursing assessment. Residents in the Main Study Hostel who were involved in the first part of the study, described above, were asked whether they had any problems with which they would like help. Also, during the use of the questionnaire and assessment tools, clinical signs and problem areas became apparent to the project nurse, a qualified district nurse. This combination of the resident's expressed need and the project nurse's professional judgement provided the link between the data collection and the intervention.

Most importantly, the interaction took place in a 'real' way; that is, it mirrored the format by which a district nurse in everyday practice would enter into an assessment of a prospective patient. If the resident expressed a need and/or if the project nurse considered that the resident needed nursing intervention, the resident was asked whether he would like to go on to the next stage. It was made quite clear to the resident that he would be helped whether or not he became part of the study. If the resident agreed that he would like to progress to the next stage, the interview continued as outlined below.

Mental Status of the Elderly Questionnaire

A proportion of the hostel residents were elderly, so it was important to assess their mental status and understanding of their environment. The Mental Status of the Aged Score is a well-validated assessment tool, being used with people over 60 years of age. It presents such questions as 'What day is it?' and 'Who is the Prime Minister?' If elderly hostel residents answered these questions incorrectly, this might have demonstrated not dementia but social isolation.

It was, however, decided that the Mental Status of the Aged Questionnaire was a useful assessment guide for the project nurse, and it was thus included in the nursing assessment, although the scores were not rigidly interpreted (Khan et al 1960). Residents in the Main

Study group, over the age of 60, were therefore asked the questions after the main questionnaire.

Recording qualitative data: explanation of comments, themes and paradigms

Rationale

Whereas it was possible to collect and collate the data in the questionnaires and validated tools as numerical values, this was neither possible nor desirable for the more complex interactions required for nursing assessment and intervention. First, such a system would have been impractical to use and would not have mirrored actual practice. Second, as had been recognized in the literature, the cumulative effect of complex nursing interventions has been demonstrated to be greater than the sum of its parts. This 'Gestalt' effect has been particularly examined by Patricia Benner, this study having adopted some of her techniques of recording as a template (Benner 1984).

More specifically, by formally engaging the project nurse in considering and recording contemporaneously events and actions, he would be 'tracking' the patient's experience (Benner 1984) and his own role within it. It would also provide insights into the nurse's problem-solving processes, particularly when recording examples of instances perceived by him as 'meaningful engagement' (Benner 1984).

Critical incident recording

The study also used techniques from phenomenological research, particularly the taking of contemporaneous notes (Flynn 1988, Patton 1990, Burnard 1991). The other technique that influenced the study has been drawn from the critical incident technique (Flanagan 1954), particularly in relation to the collection of short, significant occasions and interactions, and to their analysis to find patterns or themes in the residents' lifestyles and experiences (Dunn and Hamilton 1986). The important point regarding the use of these techniques was practical as well as investigative. The study would be taking place in 'uncharted' territory, so the exact meaning, if any, of the events as they happened might be unclear or unknown at the time. The system of recording had to be simple at the point of entry but had to enable collation and the formation of themes, with analysis at a later date.

Incident recording was taken from the theoretical framework, that is, to focus on the interactions between the men and their physical and human environment. This included their demonstrations of need, their response to services given and particularly their adaptations to these stimuli. Incidents also included examples of the men behaving as a group and the specific roles they performed within the group (Roy 1980).

District nursing intervention, for the purposes of this study, includes first, the actions of the project nurse, and second, the action taken by district nurses to whom the project nurse referred the men. To structure the project nurse's work, he kept a critical incident diary.

This study did not use the critical incident technique in the classical sense, that is, to establish high and low, or effective and less effective, standards (Norman et al 1992). It has, however, used the method of collecting qualitative data and collating it into themes.

Flanagan (1954) originally investigated the previously unknown situation of successful/unsuccessful air force pilots. By recording incidents at work either as they happened or retrospectively, essential knowledge was gained by screening for themes and patterns. Norman and Parker (1990) used this technique in an investigation on a sample similar to the one in this study when they sought the views of psychiatric patients encountering hostel life for the first time. The practical realization of this technique was achieved by the use of comments, themes and paradigms.

Comments

Comments were short sentences or phrases recorded existentially in a diary. These included the labelling of an event or an observation. Comments did not necessarily have any context at the time they were written, so they sometimes seemed disjointed. Their importance cannot, however, be underestimated. Because they were written at the time when an event or observation happened, they were an accurate portrayal of the project nurse's perception despite the complexity and confusion of everyday practice.

Themes

Comments form the basis of themes. The collection of comments and the project nurse's repeated exposure to certain incidents (such as the residents' behaviour, experience with other agencies, environmental factors, hostel circumstances and physiological and psychological factors) enabled the project nurse and the author to identify certain themes that provided an insight into the experience of the men in the sample. These themes were, at the end of the study, further classified into group themes.

It is important to emphasize at this stage that some themes were expected to emerge early on, particularly those of a physical nature, for example 'infestations', which combined with other conditions could make up a group theme of 'physical morbidity'. As the study progressed, particularly as part of the evaluation and analysis, more reflective themes would became apparent. These will be discussed in later chapters.

Paradigms

In this study, paradigms are the stories about individual men that describe a situation or interaction with health services. The paradigm was used when the whole story described a situation better than the description of its constituent parts. Paradigms were also used to exemplify themes. The main aim of the paradigm was to present a story that had created a change in the project nurse's perception (a paradigm shift) or knowledge of a particular situation.

Semi-structured interviews

This part of the assessment most closely corresponded to the nursing assessment that a district nurse would operate in practice (Baly 1981, Glasgow Caledonian University 1992). It concentrated the project nurse's attention onto possible areas in which the resident might need medical or nursing intervention. The use of the Activities of Daily Living (Roper et al 1990) as a basis for assessment is common throughout the nursing profession. It focuses the assessor's interaction with the patient onto the activities that are vital for the maintenance and promotion of a healthy, human life: breathing, eating, sleeping, mobility, temperature control, elimination, friendship, sexuality and spirituality (Roper et al 1990).

During the assessment, the project nurse continued to ask the resident what he was experiencing and what he would like done for him. This was to ensure that any interventions resulted from a collaboration between the project nurse and the resident. The project nurse was experienced in communication skills. The importance of this has been emphasized in the literature, particularly the use of 'feeding back' the resident's responses by rephrasing them and seeking affirmation.

It was also important for the project nurse to take each response as 'true' or at face value, without the use of professional or cultural assumptions, and to act accordingly. This position made an implicit acceptance that the resident might make conflicting statements at different stages in the interview or on different occasions. The project nurse treated these anomalies as a practical reality rather than as lying or a loss of good faith on the part of the resident. The nurse did not assume a complete understanding of the residents' responses or their reasons for stating them. The project nurse's function, like that of any practising nurse, was to respond to the information given and to use his experience and professional judgement, making the necessary adjustments as new information became available (Bowers 1988, Runciman 1989, Burnard 1990).

Possibility of intervention

Reflective tool used prior to intervention

The residents had their assessment and situation analysed by the project nurse using Roy's (1980) theory. This reflective tool (see Appendix I) was developed to help the project nurse to focus on the interventions necessary by reflective analysis of the assessment, recognizing that, in the literature, individuals had been observed having difficulty taking advantage of health options and making adaptations in their behaviour and lifestyle (that is, overcoming internal barriers) (Rappaport 1981, Antrobus 1987).

Using Roy's (1980) four adaptive modes as headings, the tool directs the project nurse to consider the individual resident's physical needs and problems, as well as potential problems regarding his self-worth and perception of himself as a family member and a part of society. The resident's perceptions of interdependency and loneliness are also considered (Roy 1980, Aggleton and Chalmers 1986). The project nurse wrote down his reflections regarding the information gained during the assessment in short comments; these were then developed into themes.

This study examined both whether interventions required changes to the resident's perception of his condition (overcoming possible internal barriers) by assisting the resident to act for himself (called 'resident adaptation'), as well as the effects on the individual of services and the environment (overcoming external barriers). The reflective tool was the starting place for the analysis of these, as Roy (1980) terms them, 'stimuli', which act upon the individual and promote the adaptation necessary for the individual to resolve problems.

Intervention

Treatment

The role of the project nurse, where treatment was concerned, was strictly on a 'first aid' basis or when the treatment could not be deferred (see Appendix I). The reason for this was that the project nurse's primary objective was as an agent of intervention and referral rather than as a practitioner building up a caseload. If he had routinely admitted residents, it would not have been possible to examine how the health services responded to the resident's case.

Apart from the practical benefit to the resident of treatment, this practice also served the function of creating a bond and good faith between residents and the project nurse, or as a form of entry into the individual resident's life. This function will be discussed in more detail below.

Referral

If referral was indicated following assessment, a standard letter was sent to the relevant health professional, that is, the general practitioner (GP) and where appropriate the district nurse and the community psychiatric nurse (CPN) (see Appendix II). This letter contained the following details:

- the subject's name;
- his date of birth;
- the case identification number;
- the intervention number;
- the date of the assessment;
- the reason for referral.

A copy of all referral letters was kept in the individual's intervention document.

In a small number of cases, telephone contact was also made with the practitioner involved. The criteria for this were left up to the project nurse, being based on what he would do in everyday practice and on the facilitation of the progress of his written referral.

Referrals to other statutory and voluntary agencies were made, but they were not part of the formal evaluation of this study.

Advocacy

The definition of advocacy used in this study was the project nurse acting on behalf of the resident to further his 'cause' or represent him. These acts occurred, for example, when the project nurse, as a health professional with specialist knowledge, supported an individual's application to a service or, as an articulate 'friend', accompanied a resident to an appointment. The main feature of advocacy was that these were acts that facilitated change by using the project nurse's knowledge, authority or presence, but which were not direct forms of treatments or referrals.

Evaluation

The primary focus of this study was to describe and evaluate district nursing intervention with the residents. This would comprise two distinct parts: proactivity and reactivity. First, the actions of the project nurse as a district nurse practising in a proactive manner, that is, the seeking out of the resident's health needs as the first health service contact, were described (see Appendix I). Then considered were the district nurses to whom the project nurse referred, practising in a reactive manner, that is, responding to the project nurse's referral as the second or subsequent health service contact.

Combined with this evaluation was an evaluation of the response of the GPs and CPNs, who were the other two groups of health professionals to whom the project nurse would make referrals. The evaluation of the project nurse's activities will commence in Chapter 5. What follows here is the method of evaluating the actions of the other health professionals.

Follow-up of practitioners

Between 6 and 12 weeks after the referral of the project nurse to the GPs, district nurses and/or CPNs, the author made appointments with all the practitioners and visited them. A short semi-structured interview (see Appendix I) was completed, in which the practitioners were asked what they had done in response to the referral, their rationale for any action taken and whether they considered that the referral had been appropriate. General questions were asked regarding the care of hostel-dwellers.

The expert panel

To validate and compare the action of the district nurses, who received referrals from the project nurse, six anonymized case histories of residents were prepared and presented to six district nurses from a Health Board different from the one where the study hostels were situated. These nurses were invited to an expert panel session. Presented with these six case histories, they were asked to write what they would have done had they received the referrals, their rationale and whether they thought the referral to be appropriate.

The project nurse's function was to chair a discussion of the expert panel (audiotaped and transcribed), going through each case by discussing what the panel members had written and their professional opinions. The author evaluated the data produced.

Interrater reliability checks

Interrater reliability checks were carried out by the author, the project nurse, one of the research supervisors and another nurse on parts of the the project nurse's diary. This exercise was undertaken to validate and provide contrasts on the formation and coding of themes, and will be discussed in more detail in Chapter 5.

Quantitative analysis

An extensive statistical analysis, using the computer-based Statistical Package for the Social Sciences (1990) was carried out on the data from the questionnaire and validated tools. This process has indicated some significant and highly significant relationships between factors, which will be presented and discussed in the appropriate chapters. This quantitative analysis has produced two main outcomes. First, new knowledge has been highlighted, and second, the statistical evidence has given focus and support to much of the qualitative analysis.

Qualitative analysis

Underpinning the qualitative evaluation and analysis of nursing interventions, residents' responses, the single homeless hostel environment and statutory service provision is the theoretical framework of Roy's (1980) theory (Chapter 8) and sociological analysis, including deviancy theory (Chapter 9). The framework will be used to focus the two sides of the health service–resident interaction. Both chapters will be supported by statistical and qualitative data from the study, as well as by comparisons with the literature.

Chapter 8 will present an evaluation and analysis from the perspective of the individual residents, their adaptive behaviour, barriers to health and service potential, and changes in stimuli, particularly the effect of district nursing intervention on the residents' situation. The chapter will concentrate on what the individual resident experiences and on insights into his way of living and adapting – an existential view.

Chapter 9 will present an evaluation and analysis from a societal group perspective, looking at the men as a group. Included in this will be a presentation of insights into the rationality of hostel-dwelling as a way of life, and into group and subgroup behaviours and professional assumptions made in response to the group. The chapter will concentrate on the hostel's functioning as a living organism, taking a structural view.

Separation of assessment and intervention from evaluation

Role of the author

The proposed method of assessment of the men would have involved the nurse very personally with the individual resident. Having made the assessment and conducted interventions, it would have been difficult for that nurse to make an objective evaluation of the effects of the intervention. It thus became increasingly clear that the study would need to be split into two main parts:

1. assessments (including the administration of the questionnaires, validated tools and nursing assessment) and interventions;
2. evaluation.

Need for a project nurse

It was therefore decided that a research assistant or 'project nurse' was required and that the author himself should not be involved in the assessments of, and interventions for, the men in the Main Study Hostel. The author designed and organized the study, gained access to the hostels and carried out the interviews in the Comparison Hostel. He also performed the follow-up part of the study, interviewing the practitioners to whom referrals had been made. This arrangement enabled the author to remain entirely independent of the sample in the Main Study Hostel.

Funding for the project nurse

Funding, in the form of a project grant, was gained from the Scottish Office Home and Health Department Chief Scientist's Office Health Services Research Committee for a full-time qualified district nurse who would be the project nurse for the study. A qualified district nurse was appointed to this post. He had no previous research experience. He was orientated, by the author, to the design, method and aims of the project, as well as to the staff and environment of the Main Study Hostel. It is important to state that the project nurse was directed to act as a competent district nurse in his dealings with the sample, the hostel staff and other personnel. At no time was he given any instruction regarding intervention; this was left to his own judgement. Part of the evaluation emanates from the records he kept of his actions.

Ethical principles

Two main ethical considerations emerged during the planning. The first was the recognition that the study was likely to uncover needs that would have to be addressed immediately they were discovered, whether or not they were germane to the study. This was particularly the case in the Comparison Hostel. In the Main Study Hostel, the issue would arise when a resident presented with a condition that would normally be referred but for which, because of its serious, acute nature, immediate action was necessary. These immediate interventions were therefore always carried out by the project nurse, but they did not necessarily become part of the study as some of the men needed and accepted intervention but refused to take part in the study.

Second, the project nurse would be examining patients, forming clinical judgements and making referrals within the jurisdiction of Greater Glasgow Health Board (GGHB). The study thus worked on the principle that the residents' needs came before the needs of the study, ensuring the men's right to confidentiality and to refuse to take part in the study. This did not preclude their receiving assistance if it was required. The records kept by the project nurse were stored away from the hostel in a secure file, and the information was not made available to any agency unless by prior arrangement with the resident.

The men were invited to join the study either by a face-to-face request or by written invitation. Permission to work in the hostels was gained from GDC, the Main Study Hostel owner, and, in the case of the Comparison Hostel, from the residents at one of their regular meetings. The hostels were treated by the author and project nurse as private dwellings (as opposed to public utilities) and permission to practise, received from the managers, was gained every time they attended.

The project nurse was accountable for his actions not only to the author, but also to the Community Nursing Division of GGHB Community Primary Care Unit. Once the design of the study had been formulated, ethical approval was gained from the West of Scotland Community Health Ethical Committee and professional indemnity to practise gained from the GGHB.

The fieldwork

The purpose of previous section was to demonstrate how the study took its form, to outline the decision-making processes involved and to present the design and method. This section will concentrate on the events that comprise the fieldwork. It will explain how the implementation of the research design was influenced by the day-to-day life of the hostel as well as by its organization and management. It is presented to enhance clarity. However, as with much research, events did not always occur in the order in which they are presented below.

The pilot study

During the preparatory months, the assessment and intervention document was prepared and piloted by the author in a hostel other than the Main Study Hostel. Permission was gained from GDC, the owners, to ask six residents from another large hostel in Glasgow to take part in the pilot study. It was agreed that if any of the men were found to have nursing or medical needs, the author would treat and/or refer them as necessary, but that these interventions would not be part of the evaluation.

Purpose of the pilot study

The purpose of the pilot was to test the documents for ease of use (especially with men who had communication problems), relevance to the men and time taken. Although it had been decided to use interview techniques rather than clinical screening (observations such as blood pressure and blood and urine tests) in order to gain information, it was an important function of the pilot to test the usefulness of the method chosen. Of particular interest were the validated tools, the Barthel Physical Function Index, the HAD Scale and the Mental Status in the Aged Objective Measures (Khan et al 1960, Mahoney and Barthel 1965, Zigmond and Snaith 1983).

The pilot sample

The first six men chosen, with the help of the hostel staff, comprised the pilot sample:

- Resident 1 was aged 60 and had a psychiatric history.
- Resident 2 was 76 and had a laryngectomy, but communicated by writing.
- Resident 3 had difficulty walking as well as alcohol-associated problems.
- Resident 4 was 32 years old, with a history of psychiatric problems.
- Resident 5 was aged 68 and in a wheelchair.
- Resident 6 was 82 and, although mobile, had difficulty hearing and was sometimes confused.

Findings of the pilot study

The assessment and intervention document proved easy to use. Each interview took between 30 and 60 minutes, which was as predicted. The questions were understood by the residents and appeared to elicit an accurate account of the residents' experience. The interviews were semi-structured and informal. The author sat opposite the resident, writing on the form on his lap. The resident was asked the questions in order, but if the resident wished to elaborate or talk about something else, he was allowed to do so. Most of the residents seemed to appreciate talking to someone on their own and were keen to explain how life was for them. After a few minutes, the author would gently bring the resident back to the questions.

Resident 4 did not complete the interview. He became anxious and asked to leave, and no pressure was placed on him to resume. A few days later, he approached the author and began a conversation. He said that he often became anxious with strangers and when he went to the GP. He also said that he would not mind taking part in an interview another time.

The use of interview techniques proved a helpful way of gaining information. The advantage over clinical observations was that the author was able to discover what was worrying the resident, as well as the needs perceived by the author. This enabled a satisfactory basis for referral as they involved the complete participation of the resident.

Two referrals to GPs were made as a result of the interviews. One resident was referred for urinary problems and prostatic examination, the other for an assessment of his confusion and mental status. All six residents were told how to contact the author if needed. None of them did, but the author made two subsequent visits to the hostel to see whether the referrals had been acted upon. They had, so no further intervention was taken with this group.

Problems encountered

Practical problems arose at this early stage of the fieldwork. The management at the Main Study Hostel changed, so access to the hostel had to be renegotiated with the owner and the new manager. This was time-consuming, and for a while it appeared that another hostel would have to be approached. After considerable discussion, however, the study recommenced.

There was also a serious fire at the Main Study Hostel when one of the residents fell asleep while smoking in bed. His next door neighbour was killed, the whole floor had to be abandoned, and for a short time there was speculation that the hostel would be closed. It was decided that if this were to happen, the study would follow the individual residents wherever they went. This would have been possible because some emergency arrangement would have been necessary. On a typical day in Glasgow, there are only between six and 15 hostel beds available. A cohort of over 170 men could not, therefore, have been easily absorbed into the normal admission system (GDC Hostels Unit, personal communication, 1992).

Appointment of project nurse

Division of work and rationale

During this time, the final details of the fieldwork were addressed, and the project nurse was appointed on a full-time basis for 9 months. The rationale of the division of work between the author and the project nurse centred around two principles. First, the author (the evaluator) should not be involved in any way with the Main Study group. Second, the project nurse, a district nurse, should be able to act as an autonomous practitioner, his interventions not being influenced by the author. In practice, this division worked well from the beginning as the project nurse could concentrate entirely on the Main Study Hostel, the residents and the clinical nursing aspects, while the author could concentrate on the structure and organization of the study, the negotiations, the creation of a database, evaluation and analysis. It was also assisted by the geographical distance between the Main Study Hostel and the University office (approximately 1.5 miles).

Project nurse: commencement and orientation

The project nurse started work in August 1992. He was a qualified district nurse who had been working in a neighbouring Health Board but had never before worked with homeless people or in hostels. Apart from the statutory Registration and District Nursing Diploma, he had a Diploma in Professional Studies with a speciality in communication skills.

The project nurse began his work on the study by updating his reading of the relevant literature. He was introduced to the format of the project and the staff of the Main Study Hostel, being encouraged to visit the hostel and make himself known to the men. The decision to do this emanated from the literature as well as the experience gained from the pilot work. Previous projects, whether medical, nursing or social work based, made reference to the importance of becoming known to the client group as opposed to engaging in activity 'cold' (Atkinson 1987, Burke Masters 1988, Featherstone and Ashmore 1988, El Kabir et al 1989, Heuston et al 1989). The experience of the author, particularly with resident 4 in the pilot study, had reinforced this premise.

During these preliminary visits, the project nurse started to use the critical incident diary. This took acclimatization as he mastered the technique of reporting events and interactions in short comments. He quickly organized a pattern of practice that enabled him to work and respond to the events in the hostel but ensured that they were recorded. This was based around the use of short-term (2- or 3-hour) sessions in the hostel, followed by recording.

The project nurse piloted the assessment and intervention document with 10 residents of the Main Study Hostel. This procedure was to ensure that he understood the study and the documents, and that the author and project nurse understood one another. The project nurse found that each interview took approximately an hour. These first 10 men were interviewed during the course of 1 week. As no difficulties or flaws were discovered, these 10 residents were included in the Main Study sample.

The assessment and intervention period

The project nurse worked in the Main Study Hostel recruiting and interviewing residents for a period of 11 weeks, excluding holidays. The author began the data collection at the Comparison Hostel 6 weeks after the project nurse began collecting data in the Main Study Hostel, and continued for a period of 5 weeks.

An attempt was made to interview all the 170 residents of the Main Study Hostel. It was expected that approximately 50 residents would require some form of intervention. At first, the project nurse relied on opportunistic encounters with the residents in the communal areas of the hostel. These included the two day rooms, the foyer and the refectory. This technique produced a number of interviews. After a few weeks, letters of invitation were distributed to the residents' rooms, this being repeated towards the end of the study. This pattern of practice will be discussed further in Chapter 5.

Venue

The interviews in the Main Study Hostel took place in a small room off the main foyer, which was designated as a first aid room but was commonly used as a broom cupboard. It contained two chairs and an old couch as well as a sink. It was decided that the project nurse would wear a white uniform tunic to emphasize his presence as a district nurse. He put a notice on the door when he was in the hostel and continued to work in sessions. This ensured that he was operating at maximum concentration when undertaking interviews. He would generally undertake no more than four interviews in one session.

Effects on data-gathering of alcohol use by residents

As the study progressed, the project nurse adapted the times he attended, but in general most of his sessions occurred on weekdays. He tended not to work there on Thursdays as it was 'Giro day', when men received their benefits. Some men would drink excessive amounts of alcohol and stay around the communal areas of the hostel; the resulting atmosphere proved unconducive to effective interviewing.

However, the project nurse made no hard and fast rules about residents being 'dry' when he saw them. If a man was obviously drunk, he would always speak with him, but he would only interview when the resident appeared in a more sober state. This was an important distinction not only for the reliability of the information collected, but also for the resident's well-being. Decisions regarding intervention were better taken when the resident had a full understanding of what was happening.

Safety

Regard was also given to the safety of the project nurse. Violence is often seen in hostels; this had been experienced by the author and others working in the field. Such situations commonly arise from only slight provocation and can escalate to sometimes life-threatening proportions in seconds.

The project nurse was qualified in communication skills. His manner was at all times non-confrontational. Thus, he sought not to challenge conflicting information from a resident but to record it. This policy went in tandem with the theoretical part of the design described above. The project nurse was also directed to leave any violent situation immediately, making no attempt to resolve the situation by himself.

These safety measures were not based on an assumption that this hostel was always violent or that homeless men are more violent than other people: it was simply a practical recognition that violence does occur. During the study, the project nurse was not involved in any violent events, although violence did occur between and to various residents.

Confidentiality

During the study, the project nurse maintained confidentiality with respect to the residents' information. The case notes were brought back to the University office each day and kept in a locked filing cabinet. A certain amount of liaison took place with the hostel staff, but neither side exchanged specific clinical information. Apart from ethical considerations, there was also a practical benefit to the care with which the information was treated: it appeared to increase trust between the project nurse and the residents.

Liaison of the project nurse with the author

The project nurse and the author met on most days at their office in the University. As mentioned earlier, the author did not influence the assessments or interventions, but he did advise on methods of recording so that notes were mutually understood. The project nurse would sometimes seek an exchange of views on what constituted 'normal' nursing practice in particular instances, although residents were not mentioned by name. This kind of discussion is normal among nurses in practice, particularly when district nurses meet together after their visits. The issue was resolved, as far as the study was concerned, by the project nurse recording any action he took that he considered would be unusual or outside normal nursing practice.

Comparison Hostel

To gain access to the Comparison Hostel, the author met with officials at the GDC Hostels Unit. They offered a hostel of comparable size to the Main Study Hostel. The author was directed to attend a residents' meeting to inform them about the study and to gain their permission to recruit and interview. This was received on condition that the appropriate referrals were made if necessary and that recruiting took place in the communal areas only, no approaches being made to the men in their rooms. This was counted as fair by all parties, taking into account that the men in the Comparison Hostel were helping the study with little direct return for their involvement, that is, they were only answering questionnaires and not receiving the service of a full nursing assessment with intervention.

The interviews in the Comparison Hostel took place in a number of venues. Each resident was asked whether he wanted to be interviewed in private. If he did, an empty sitting room or quiet area was found. However, most did not want to move from the main television room and were quite happy to speak there. The room offered some privacy as it was large and busy, so that it was possible to have a private conversation without being overheard. The interviews took between 20 and 40 minutes.

Timescale

The completion time of the recruiting and interviewing in both hostels was decided by scrutiny of the resident list. As far as possible, the study was trying to 'capture' a group of residents as they were at a particular point in time, so that there would be a representative mix of short-stay and long-stay residents. If the study had carried on indefinitely, 170 interviews might have been possible in the Main Study Hostel and 220 in the Comparison Hostel. This would mainly have comprised new residents 'topping up' the number and would have distorted the results.

In addition, there would still have been a large group of men who would not take part. An important part of the study was to demonstrate a lack of co-operation as well as active participation.

The recruiting of residents in the Comparison Hostel gave the author an opportunity to observe the hostel and its men as a potential place for district nurses to practise on a regular basis. It appeared that many of the men needed help but did not respond to the author's presence. In particular, there were a number of very frail elderly men. Active case-finding certainly appeared to be successful with some men. However, many others appeared to be suspicious of newcomers, and it seemed to the author that these men would be more likely to respond over a longer period of time. The hostel staff agreed with this observation.

An evaluation and analysis of the number of men recruited, assessed and receiving intervention will be outlined in Chapters 5 and 10. At this point, however, it is interesting to point out that a high number of interventions took place in the first few weeks.

In the Comparison Hostel, 100 interviews took place using the criteria set by the hostel staff. By the end of the 5-week period, the author had approached all the men he had encountered in the communal areas, numbering approximately 190. One terminally ill man was seen in his room, as were three others who specifically invited the author to come in (one with the offer of a dram – which was not accepted!).

Both author and project nurse found it very difficult to set a particular number of interviews to be achieved in a day. The most important action was, where possible, to attend in each hostel every day during the period. The regular appearance of the author and project nurse had a positive effect on recruitment as the men in both hostels became used to the presence of the author or project nurse. Nevertheless, both author and project nurse experienced days when no interviews were forthcoming.

Other activities

During the early part of the fieldwork, a request for assistance was received from the Tuberculosis Surveillance Unit at the GGHB, the author and project nurse being asked to help to organize as many residents as possible to attend for radiographic screening. The men were to receive a money voucher for attendance at the Unit, approximately a mile away, and to be given an appropriate appointment at the hospital outpatient department when necessary. The author and project nurse assisted the hostel staff in notifying the men, and 97 men attended the Surveillance Unit.

Although this was not a formal part of the project, the large response from the men was worthy of note. The author collected information from the Surveillance Unit staff that proved relevant to the study and will be discussed in Chapters 5 and 8.

The project nurse's activities until the end of the study

The recruitment, interviews and intervention in the Main Study Hostel lasted from September 1992 until January 1993. After that time, the project nurse continued to visit the hostel on a part-time basis. The purpose of this activity was to keep in touch with the progress of individual men and to consolidate the findings of the fieldwork.

This gave the project nurse the opportunity to spend time with the residents that was not preoccupied with completing assessments. The literature had shown that spending a period of time with people for no specific reason, or for a variety of reasons, as opposed to allotting a limited section of time for a particular appointment or purpose, is a valuable part of nursing practice (Bishop and Scudder 1990).

For the project nurse, the period after the main recruitment and intervention was used to clarify the process of formulating themes and paradigms.

Author's activities

The author was engaged in interviewing the medical and nursing personnel to whom the referrals had been made. In a semi-structured interview (see Appendix I), they were asked questions regarding their actions following the referral, how they had come to their decisions, any difficulties they had encountered, how well they found the resident to be, the appropriateness of the referral and their previous experience with homeless men. This process was time-consuming as visits had to be made in various parts of the large city of Glasgow, and none of the GPs offered separate business appointments. Visits had, in the main, to be made at the close of their surgeries.

Although a considerable amount of time was spent waiting, this aspect of the study proved fruitful, only one GP refusing to see the author. An evaluation of this process will take place in Chapter 6.

The expert panel

The expert panel was formed from district nurses from a neighbouring Health Board. They were invited to meet on a Saturday afternoon in a neutral setting (a meeting room in a local church), presented with the six anonymized case histories and asked to indicate what their action would be if they were to be given a similar referral. After writing down their comments, they took part in a tape-recorded discussion session, which was subsequently transcribed. The event was chaired by the project nurse, although the author was in attendance. The session went as expected. (See Chapter 7 for a full discussion.)

Conclusion

This chapter has shown how the study was organized and implemented, the results and evaluation being discussed in later chapters. In a study of this kind, where the author and project nurse were working in a particularly challenging area, it was expected that there would be difficulties. However, despite some of the difficulties mentioned, the study progressed very much as planned. No changes to the design were necessary after the commencement of the fieldwork part of the study.

Chapter 4 will present the first part of the results, concentrating on the data gained from the questionnaires administered in both hostels, and comparing and contrasting them.

Chapter 4
Results: Part 1

The focus of this chapter is the presentation of the data gathered in the questionnaire administered to the samples in both hostels (see Appendix I). The chapter will describe the results by placing the study into a demographic context encompassing the other hostels in Glasgow and their residents. An outline of the patterns of recruitment used by the author and project nurse to gain access to the men will be presented. The hostels' residents will be described using the results of the questionnaires, statistically significant relationships and contrasts between the hostels.

Hostel accommodation in Glasgow

Table 4.1 lists the permanent hostels in Glasgow. It is difficult to establish exactly how many individual men use the hostels. However, the Glasgow District Council Single Person's Section keeps records of how many men and women are admitted to hostels every year and of the number who leave.

The admissions and discharges of the Council-run hostels are presented in Table 4.2, giving some indication of the turnover and number of individuals using the service. An unknown number are admitted more than once, especially if they have been evicted (usually for violent or unruly behaviour), have short periods in prison or hospital, or lead a transient lifestyle.

The study hostels

The Main Study Hostel

From information gained from the owner of the hostel, as well as from other personal contact with older Glaswegians who had attended the school that was next door, the author discovered that the Great Eastern Hotel had been built in 1907 as a residence for the employees of

Table 4.1: Hostel provision in Glasgow

Male hostels	Owners	Total Beds
Peter McCann House (Pilot hostel)	Glasgow Housing Department	254
James Duncan House (Comparison hostel)	Glasgow Housing Department	252
Great Eastern Hotel (Main study hostel)	Commercially run	170[a]
Robertson House	Glasgow Housing Department	254
Laidlaw House	Glasgow Housing Department	248
Bellgrove Hotel	Commercially run	250[b]
Mixed Hostel		
Norman Street Hostel	Glasgow Housing Department (with 31 female beds)	70
Female Hostels		
Jean Morris House	Glasgow Housing Department	48
Hope House	Salvation Army	73
	Total male beds	1489
	Total female beds	152
	All beds	1641

[a] The original complement was 300 beds but only 170 were in use.
[b] Approximate number because access was denied.

Table 4.2: Admissions and discharges in Glasgow District Council-run hostels 1993

Age (years)	Admissions	Discharges
18–21	740	297
22–24	481	235
25–30	796	159
31–40	729	604
41–50	496	323
51–60	323	891
60+	139	0
Total	3704	2509

Beds: 1189 male/female; 1028 male only

Anderson's Mill. Its role gradually changed over the next 30 years to that of a general working men's hostel. However, after World War II and the subsequent decline of the traditional heavy industries and increase in unemployment, its role again changed to that of a hostel for the homeless, in which the majority of the residents are unemployed and rely on state benefits for their income.

The hostel has five storeys, only three of which are currently in use as the roof and fourth and fifth floors required extensive repair work as a result of flooding. Part of the second floor was damaged by fire in September 1991. There are currently no plans to repair the roof or the fire-damaged area. The hostel can accommodate up to 250 residents, although there are generally between 120 and 170 in residence.

Facilities

At the time of the study, each floor had central toilet and washing facilities (although a few minor alterations have been made since the study). These areas included showers (none of which worked), several sinks, a urinal and toilet cubicles. There were further washing facilities in the basement, where four baths were to be found.

There were no cooking facilities and very limited access to power points for boiling water and so on. On the ground floor, there was a dining room where breakfast was provided between 6.30 and 8.00 am. Lunch and dinner were not provided. On the ground floor there were a common room with one pool table and a TV room.

Staffing

During the day, the following staff were generally on duty:

- the manager and/or assistant manager (neither of whom worked during the evening or at the weekend);
- one or two hostel workers;
- two or three porters (some being residents);
- three cleaners;
- one kitchen worker;
- one laundry worker.

In the evenings, a hostel worker and three porters were on duty. At night, one hostel worker was generally on duty.

Statutory services

During the period of the study, one **district nurse** visited fortnightly.

A **community psychiatric nursing service** had been set up at the time of the study, which dealt exclusively with the hostel residents. This service has recently been expanded by employing a staff nurse and a care assistant to work with the community psychiatric nurse (CPN) already in post.

There are two **health centres** within 1 mile of the hostel, where residents can visit a GP. Most of the residents were registered at the larger centre.

In terms of **social work** input, Strathclyde Social Work Department provided a 'peripatetic team', a home help-type service to identify mainly elderly hostel-dwellers. In addition, a special Homeless Team was located a mile away, dealing with residents and their housing and benefit needs.

Voluntary services

The **British Red Cross Society** offered a bathing service every Saturday morning. This had been instigated 2 years before the study by a Red Cross worker (Donaghue 1989).

In addition to this, a **lay preacher** visited the hostel every Wednesday evening to hold a service and distribute tea and biscuits.

The Comparison Hostel

The Comparison Hostel had been purpose built in the 1970s, so the fabric of the building and the facilities were in a much better condition than those of the Main Study Hostel.

Facilities

There were rooms on the ground floor for disabled residents, and a residents' lift was available. All the showers and washing facilities were in good working order, so it was possible for the men to keep clean if they wished.

Staffing

The staffing quota was much higher than in the Main Study Hostel. There were more staff at every level (about 10 on the day shift), enabling residents to receive greater attention.

Statutory services

The statutory services had the same access and operated in the same manner as in the Main Study Hostel.

Patterns of recruiting to the study

The Main Study Hostel

Number of residents

At the start of the study, there were 177 men living at the Great Eastern Hotel. By the end of the study, there were 162.

The sample

During the study, the project nurse was able to gain information on 168 residents (although for some, only their name, age and length of stay at the hostel were available). Of these, 106 were interviewed.

During the first week of fieldwork, the nursing assessments commenced, 11 being carried out during this week. Over the next 10 weeks, 95 assessments were carried out, giving a total of 106 residents who were assessed. Of these, 87 were still in residence at the end of the study.

In the first 2 weeks of the study, almost all of those assessed required intervention from the project nurse. During the third week, a drop in both the assessment and the intervention rates was observed. Up until the end of the second week, there had been 40 assessments and 33 interventions. By the end of the third week, this had increased to only 47 assessments and 36 interventions.

It was considered important, by both author and project nurse, to try to improve recruitment by making sure that all the residents knew about the study. A written invitation to those residents living on the first floor was distributed at the beginning of the fourth week, and as a result, a moderate increase in assessment rate was achieved. The project nurse also attended twice in the early morning and twice in the evening to improve recruitment. By the halfway point in the sixth week, 72 assessments and 45 interventions had been carried out.

A significant drop in the assessment and intervention rates took place between the seventh and ninth weeks, prompting the issuing of a second letter, this time to those living on the second and third floors. This had a short-lived effect and was followed up by a final letter in the tenth week, targeting those yet to be assessed living on all three floors. A summary of this pattern of recruiting is provided in Table 4.3.

From a practice point of view, it is worth noting that half the interventions took place within the first 3 weeks and that nearly three-quarters had taken place by the end of the seventh week. This will be discussed in Chapter 10.

Table 4.3: Pattern of assessments and interventions

Methods of recruitment (Main study hostel)	Number of residents
Assessment interviews followed by interventions	67
Assessment interview not followed by intervention	39
Total interviews	106
Resident approaches and opportunistic encounters by project nurse	92
Letters to residents floor by floor: First floor (week 3) Second floor (week 9) Third floor (week 10)	34
Recruitment made by evening and early morning shift	12

The Comparison Hostel

Number of residents

During the time the author undertook the interviews, 227 residents were living at the Comparison Hostel.

The sample

During the fieldwork, the author was able to gain information on all 227 residents (for some, only their name and age being available). Of these, 180 were approached for interviews, 100 of whom participated in the interviews. Of these, three did not complete the interview.

The demographic profile of the hostel

The data were obtained through answers to a structured questionnaire containing 26 questions and the scores derived from questionnaires concerning physical function (the Barthel Index), mental state (the Hospital Anxiety and Depression Scale, HAD), and the effects on the individual's life of alcohol use and the amount of smoking.

Comparison of hostels: limitations of the analysis

Where appropriate, tables will be presented demonstrating statistically significant positive relationships between hostels ($p = <0.001$). Readers who are interested in the full set of tables containing details of all the frequencies in both hostels may refer to the author or to the original thesis (Atkinson 1997). The following points regarding the tables of comparison must be emphasized at this stage:

- Using the structured questionnaire, 106 men were interviewed in the Main Study Hostel and 100 men in the Comparison Hostel. The men, in both hostels, were specifically recruited neither as identified individuals nor as comparative matched pairs created for the study (this being considered by the author and others as being too unwieldy in already difficult circumstances). There is no claim, therefore, that they are representative of the population of single homeless men in Glasgow or Scotland.
- Of the men who took part in the interviews, not all answered every question. In particular, some of the older, frailer men found it difficult to concentrate and focus on some of the questions. This factor may have influenced the results.
- This study does not, therefore, make major claims as a result of the comparison of hostels in this chapter. Statistically significant comparisons are only presented if, in the author's view, they present an insight into the residents' health, lifestyle, environment and aspirations.

In this chapter, the following measures have been taken to ensure that only relevant comparisons are used:

1. Only comparisons with a statistical significance of p = <0.001 are used.
2. Of these, only comparisons that have other supporting evidence are presented. Tables containing non-significant data from the two hostels are presented when the frequencies of variables and values are discussed.
3. The hostel comparisons are used only for discussion and in an attempt to promote understanding. They are not used to form the recommendations outlined in Chapter 10.

Age of residents

There was one variable for which information was gained on all the residents in both hostels, namely age. This proved very useful as a statistical comparison showed no significant difference between the two groups.

There was a higher number of younger men in the Comparison Hostel. This may be accounted for by the fact that the hostel is commonly used as a place of emergency accommodation by the Glasgow District Council Homeless Unit for men in crisis. The Main Study Hostel was a place of self-referral rather than part of a formal admission process. Men tended to come to the Main Study Hostel from other hostels or homeless situations, whereas many of the young men arriving at the Comparison Hostel had less experience of being homeless.

Because the variable of age involved all the residents, a further comparison was made between the group of men from both hostels who took part in the interviews and those who did not. No statistical difference was established, although there was a slightly higher number of men under 25 years among those interviewed.

Marital status of residents

There was no statistically significant difference between the two groups in terms of marital status. It should be pointed out that the term 'single' is somewhat ambivalent. Some of the men had been in a long-term relationship or were in an 'on/off' relationship with one woman. As they had never been formally married, they could not be divorced, so they described themselves as single.

A few were currently in a relationship but lived separately from their partner and children in order that the woman could receive benefits as a single mother. A colloquial distinction is made in Glasgow between a man who generally lives with his partner (called by some a 'bidey in') and a man who stays only from time to time (a 'kippy in'). The point of this description is to demonstrate that there were variations in and nuances of long- and short-term relationships apparent in both hostels, and these were not adequately gleaned by the questionnaire.

It is interesting to note the relatively large number of widowed men (12) in the Main Study Hostel. The author attempted to place this number in the context of the local population, but this was not possible in any meaningful way. However, if the author, while practising as a district nurse, had a caseload of 50–60 patients, he would normally expect to have only one or two widowers to visit. It appears that hostels might be a place of choice for a significant number of widowers, which may indicate the lack of other more appropriate communal accommodation. This possible lack of accommodation will be referred to again in Chapter 10.

Residents' length of stay in their hostels

There was an appreciable difference between the two groups with regard to this variable. A statistically significant relationship was found but discarded because the sample from the Main Study Hostel constituted nearly all that hostel's population, whereas only limited information was available from the Comparison Hostel. The comparison sample showed a larger percentage of men who had been resident under

1 year, although the Main Study Hostel sample had more men who had been resident for between 1 and 5 years.

This difference may be affected by two factors. First, the Comparison Hostel was the designated admission hostel for the Council-run hostel system. Men would go there first before being transferred elsewhere. Second, some of the more recent residents in the Comparison Hostel appeared to congregate around the communal areas. A number of the residents who had been there for longer kept themselves to their rooms or spent much of the day outside the hostel. The author, who interviewed the Comparison sample, was not permitted to seek out residents in their rooms as the questionnaire, by itself, was considered to be without therapeutic value by the management (unlike the situation in the Main Study Hostel, where nursing intervention was enacted).

Residents' length of stay in homeless accommodation and time since they lived with their families

There was no significant difference between the two groups regarding the length of time since residents had lived with their families and their length of stay in hostel accommodation.

The residents who had recently come into hostel accommodation had, in the main, recently lived with their families. However, 10 residents had resided in homeless accommodation for 6 years or more but had lived with their families within the past 5 years. In addition, 20 men who had been in hostel accommodation for less than 1 year had lived away from their families for longer than that period. This evidence supports the previous assertion that some men move in and out of hostels and their family home, and that some men appear to become detached from their families some time before they come into hostel accommodation.

As expected, the Chi-square test showed a statistically significant relationship between the two variables of length of stay in homeless accommodation and time since the men had lived with their families (Table 4.4). What is interesting, however, is that only half of the men (21) who had been resident in hostels for under a year had lived with their families immediately before admission. Similarly, 16 out of the 49 men who had been resident for between 1 and 5 years had last stayed with their families 6 or more years before.

From a nursing practice point of view, these nuances of hostel use proved illuminating, particularly with regard to the possible health-care needs of men who become detached from their families, become physically and/or mentally dysfunctional and gravitate into homeless accommodation. In Chapter 7, the relationship between this pattern

Table 4.4: Residents' (from both hostels) length of stay in homeless accommodation compared with the last time they lived with their family.

| Length of stay | Last time resident with family | | | | |
	Under 1 year	1–5 years	6+ years	Never	Total
Under 1 year	21	11	9	1	42
1–5 years	4	29	16	0	49
6 + years	3	7	71	2	83
Total	28	47	96	3	174

Chi–squared test, $p = <0.001$.

and mental illness will be demonstrated, and in Chapter 10 the implications for patterns of nursing practice will be highlighted.

Employment history

Of the men interviewed, five men were in employment. A discussion with the hostel staff confirmed the low number of men in work. Apart from the general problems of unemployment and factors such as poor physical and mental health, with associated features such as excessive alcohol use and poor personal hygiene, the men in employment told the author and project nurse that having a hostel as a home address often mitigated against the chance of finding a job. It seemed to the men that this had a negative influence on their success.

Residents registered with a general practitioner, distance and treatment pattern

In the Main Study Hostel, nearly all the residents were registered with a general practitioner (GP). In the Comparison Hostel, this information was not kept, but 91 out of the 96 men who answered the question were registered with a GP. The hostel manager considered that most men were on a GP's list. She knew this because staff often had to help residents to register and/or to obtain medical attention for them.

Most of the men lived within a mile of their GP's surgery. The Main Study Hostel and the Comparison Hostel were near the largest health centre in Glasgow and another health centre based in the Royal Infirmary. A high percentage of men were currently receiving treatment from their GP. In many cases, this involved collecting repeat prescriptions and/or sickness certificates.

The majority of men who answered the question had seen their GP within the previous 3 months. In Chapter 10, the possibilities of this contact as an opportunity for assessment and monitoring by the primary health-care team will be discussed.

Hospital admissions history

Half of those who answered in the Main Study Hostel and the Comparison Hostel had been admitted to hospital in the previous 2 years. This result indicates the high degree of morbidity found in both samples. Most of the admissions were for physical illness, multiple admissions occurring in a third of cases in the Main Study Hostel and nearly a quarter of cases in the Comparison Hostel.

The significance of these patterns will be discussed in later chapters, particularly with regard to residents with a hospital admission history, and to those who feel unwell and refer themselves to a health professional.

Admission to hospital for mental illness

Fifteen men in the Main Study Hostel and 13 of the men in the Comparison Hostel had been in a mental hospital within the previous 5 years. This demonstrates that a number of men had a mental illness history. There was no evidence that a large number of men were being discharged straight into hostel accommodation from mental hospitals. However, it must again be emphasized that the study did not reach all the men in the hostels.

From the evidence of the men in the interviews, as well as from hostel and welfare staff, it appeared that a number of men were discharged from hospital into suitable housing and then, at a later stage, became residents of a hostel following illness or the breakdown of their housing circumstances.

Current attendance at an outpatient clinic

Eleven men in each hostel sample were currently attending outpatient clinics, mainly for physical conditions. One man from the Main Study Hostel and three from the Comparison Hostel were attending an outpatient department for diagnosed mental illness.

Nursing visits to the hostels

Four men in the Main Study Hostel and 3 in the Comparison Hostel had been seen by a district nurse, from a local health centre, during their stay in their hostel. Five men in the Main Study Hostel and 4 in the Comparison Hostel had been seen by a CPN from the dedicated hostel team. Only one district nurse was currently visiting in the Main Study Hostel. The visiting patterns of nurses are discussed in Chapter 6.

Visits to the accident and emergency (A & E) department

The Chi-square test demonstrated a significant difference between the two hostels in the pattern of residents' visits to accident and emergency (A and E), a result that was highly significant (Table 4.5). It should be noted that the Main Study Hostel was situated closer to the hospital (Glasgow Royal Infirmary) than the Comparison Hostel. Historically, that is, before the establishment of the nearest health centre, built in the early 1980s, a large number of men from the Main Study Hostel used the Infirmary.

Table 4.5: Residents' visits to A&E within the previous 2 years.

| Visits | Number of residents | |
	Main study hostel	Comparison hostel
None	36	69
One	18	12
Two	7	8
More than two	24	4
Total	85	93

Chi-squared test, $p = < 0.001$.

Prison record

Half of the sample in the Main Study Hostel and half of that in the Comparison Hostel had been in prison. In the Main Study Hostel, over a third had been in prison more than twice. The author and project nurse found that many of these men were sent to prison on a regular basis, often connected with drinking offences.

Feelings of health and illness

'How do you feel?' proved to be one of the most successful questions in the study. When the author first considered using the question, several practitioners thought that the men would tend to say 'Not well' in order to gain attention from health professionals, but this proved far from the case. The majority of men felt well and said so. It seemed that if they did not feel well, they were also honest, as the feeling of being unwell was supported by some evidence from other variables, particularly feelings of health compared with hospital admission history, although this relationship was not statistically significant.

About half the men who, in the project nurse's view, needed intervention said that they did not feel well or that they felt ill. In addition,
high levels of anxiety and depression, and the use of the A and E
department, were seen among men who did not feel well. Perhaps the
most uplifting feature of this evidence is that from an intensive, time-
consuming study, the author and project nurse, as nurses, discovered
the value of asking the patient 'How do you feel?'

Living preferences

Two-thirds of the sample in the Main Study Hostel and a similar
number of the Comparison sample preferred to live in a house or flat,
but a sizeable minority (about a third in each hostel) preferred to live in
hostel accommodation.

Approximately half the men wished to live by themselves, but,
conversely, another group preferred company. A contrast between the
hostels may be seen. Although the largest group in the Main Study
Hostel wanted to live alone, nearly a third of them wanted to live with
their wife and/or family.

The author and project nurse found that men who had lived in
hostels for many years but wanted to live with their families tended to
see their lifestyle as aberrant or dysfunctional. Conversely, other men,
who had only lived in hostels for a short time, would be reasonably
happy with their lot and considered themselves to be living a 'normal'
lifestyle. This issue will be discussed in more detail in Chapter 9.

As with the simple question 'How do you feel?', the question
'Where is home?' provided great insight into the men's experience. The
largest group of men did not consider either the Main Study Hostel or
their family home to be home, compared with over half of the men in
the Comparison sample. The Chi-square test showed this difference to
be statistically significant (Table 4.6). A large number in both groups
considered their hostel as home. When the author and project nurse

Table 4.6: Residents' perception of where 'home' was.

Where is home?	Main study hostel	Comparison hostel
In the hostel	35	35
Family birthplace	16	50
Elsewhere	40	8
Total	91	93

Chi-squared test, $p = < 0.001$.

asked the men this question, some were found to answer that although they would have liked to live with their families, they considered their hostel as home. This adaptation appeared to stem from a pragmatic appreciation of their circumstances.

Functional status as assessed by the Barthel Index

At the beginning of the fieldwork in the Main Study Hostel, the Barthel Index appeared to be of limited use as an indicator of the men's physical function. Almost all of the men scored 100, indicating full physical function. The project nurse reported that although this presented a relatively accurate picture of what the men's physical capabilities were, it did not express the effort required to achieve the tasks; that is, some men could undertake all the tasks listed in the Index, such as walking, grooming and so on, but spent 15 minutes walking up the stairs for example, or took a long time to get to the toilet. Because there were no lifts and a limited number of toilets, the men living in the Main Study Hostel had no choice but to persevere.

These issues were brought into sharp relief when the fieldwork began in the Comparison Hostel. It then became apparent that the Barthel Index scores of the Comparison sample demonstrated that it was possible to live in the Comparison Hostel with a lower level of physical function. Thus, the Barthel Index was also acting as an indicator of the hostels' facilities and ability to cater for disabled residents. The Comparison Hostel had better facilities than the Main Study Hostel (a lift and rooms on ground floor). This enabled residents with varying degrees of physical dysfunction (one in a wheelchair, another with multiple sclerosis, one with a fractured tibia and one who was terminally ill and *in extremis*) to live in the Comparison Hostel. The rather brutal conclusion that may be drawn from this analysis was that for residents to be able to function in the Main Study Hostel, they needed to have a high level of physical ability.

This was borne out by the experience of the author and project nurse, who noticed that frail residents would exist on a 'narrow edge' of being able to function physically and independently for sometimes long periods. When they became ill, however, they tended to deteriorate very quickly. The terminally ill man in the Comparison Hostel, who scored zero on the Barthel Index, had been physically independent 2 weeks before. Because of the better facilities in the Comparison Hostel, he was able to remain there until he died. In the Main Study Hostel, men tended to be sent to hospital whenever their condition deteriorated, although this did not always result in admission. The project nurse witnessed one physically dysfunctional resident who was seen in and discharged from A and E three times before he was finally admitted to hospital, the outcome his GP had been attempting to achieve.

To summarize, the Barthel Index proved a useful tool as it both demonstrated the individual's physical function and, unexpectedly, acted as an indicator of the hostels' facilities and their effect on physically dysfunctional residents, particularly their ability to remain in hostel accommodation.

HAD Scale

Anxiety

The HAD Scale (Zigmond and Snaith 1983) has been used in research conducted in community settings (Snaith, personal communication, 1993) but not with homeless men. Some health-care professionals with whom the author spoke were doubtful about the use of the tool with this group. They suspected that the men might give a particular answer in order to gain attention. This notion was, however, disproved in this study. Approximately half of the Main Study sample fell within the normal range, as did two-thirds in the Comparison Hostel. The important feature of a high anxiety score is that, unlike a high depression score, it is susceptible to environmental factors. Chapter 7 outlines further evidence, provided by Dr R.P. Snaith, as an expert witness, regarding the significance of the HAD Scale results of this study.

Depression

Again, it will be observed in Table 4.7 that the results of the majority of the men in the Comparison Hostel fell within the normal range, but those of only just under a third of the sample from the Main Study Hostel did. A quarter of the men at the Main Study Hostel fell within

Table 4.7: Hospital Anxiety and Depression Scale.

| | Number of residents | |
Scores	Main study hostel	Comparison hostel
0–6	31	61
7–9	28	16
10–21	22	9
Total	81	86

Chi-squared test, p = <0.001.
Scores: 0–6 = normal range; 7–9 = intermediate range; 10–21 = high range.

the high range compared with about a tenth of the Comparison Hostel sample. The Chi-square test demonstrated this to be statistically significant.

The express purpose of the depression tool is to isolate treatable clinical, biogenic depression by identifying anhedonia, a loss of the ability to experience pleasure. Biogenic depression is not specifically susceptible to environmental factors or to alcohol use. Thus, whereas a poor environment and/or a history of alcohol abuse may increase an individual's anxiety, these are not causal factors in biogenic depression.

This was borne out by a comparison of these variables, which showed no statistical relationship. Residents with a high depression score were found to be equally distributed throughout the impact of alcohol and length of stay comparisons. The occurrence, in the general population, of this form of non-reactive depression is approximately 5% or less (Snaith, personal communication, 1993). The level of high depression scores in both hostels (approximately 25% in the Main Study Hostel and 10% in the Comparison Hostel) is, therefore, great, especially in the Main Study Hostel. This discovery became one of the most important findings of the study.

Impact of alcohol on lifestyle

The purpose of the use of the Impact of Alcohol on Lifestyle Questionnaire was an attempt to measure the effects of alcohol rather than simply the amount of consumption. This proved useful, and the scores were supported when compared with other variables, particularly anxiety and prison record. Over half the men in the Main Study Hostel sample scored within the two higher score levels compared with just under half of those in the Comparison Hostel sample. These show a very high impact of alcohol on both populations. It is, however, important to point out that not all the men drank alcohol or drank it to excess, and whereas alcohol use is an important factor with these homeless men, generalization to the population of homeless men would not be supported by these results.

Drug use

Several of the younger residents (under 25 years of age) used illegal substances, either by injection, orally or by smoking. Some of these younger men did not drink alcohol, some even being highly critical of the use of alcohol. Three of the under-25-year-olds in the Main Study Hostel and 7 in the Comparison Hostel admitted to the author and project nurse that they used drugs. Not everyone was, however, willing to discuss this issue.

Smoking

A minority of each sample smoked more than 20 cigarettes daily. The author and project nurse were constantly told by residents that the number of cigarettes smoked was controlled by their cost rather than by any health consideration.

Summary and conclusion

The results from the questionnaire and validated tools, together with the statistical analysis, proved useful and highly productive. The comparison of the two hostels was especially worthwhile. Demographic factors such as age, marital status, employment history and prison record were found to be comparable. It was not possible to 'prove' statistically that the Main Study Hostel sample was representative or typical of all the hostel residents or of single homeless men because of the number of non-responses, but the comparison was a success as it assisted the author to gain knowledge about the Main Study Hostel and its population.

The differences between the hostels discussed in this chapter have no significance for the subsequent nursing assessments in the intervention stage or for the analysis that follows in the remaining chapters. These chapters will focus on the comparison between different variables, for example between the level of high depression scores and residents' perceptions of their circumstances.

The contrasts described in this chapter enabled an analysis to take place giving insights into the life experience of the hostel samples as a whole and detailing specific differences between the two samples. Particular relationships were highlighted, especially in association with anxiety and depression, use of the health services, prison record, impact of alcohol and adaptive patterns over the length of stay. These will be examined in later chapters.

Perhaps most importantly for the author was that the results described in this chapter began to demonstrate that the residents' experience and perception of their life in the hostels could be examined in both a group and an individual context. On the one hand, some men felt 'at home' in the hostels, their lifestyle appeared more settled and they had companionship. On the other hand, others demonstrated loneliness, anxiety and poor health, and were certainly not settled in their hostel. This was the first time that statistical evidence and a demographic profile had been used to gain specific and complex information regarding the residents.

The individual experience and the qualitative findings will begin to be examined in Chapter 5 and will concentrate on the results of the evidence gathered by the project nurse, particularly during the intervention phase of the study. The experience of the men as a group (and as subgroups) will be examined in more detail in Chapter 9.

Chapter 5
Results: Part 2

The previous chapter concentrated on a demographic profile relating to the residents of the Main Study Hostel and the Comparison Hostel. The profile of the men and the hostel in which they lived indicated the context in which the activities of the project nurse, as a district nurse, were conducted, that is, the context within which he made appropriate interventions with the sample subjects in the Main Study Hostel.

This chapter will describe the nursing assessment and the planning for intervention, particularly the use of the reflective tool developed from Roy's (1980) theory and model (Aggleton and Chalmers 1986). The project nurse's diary, recording comments, which led to the themes and paradigms, is also described in this chapter.

The chapter will demonstrate patterns and types of proactive district nursing intervention, that is, the project nurse going into an environment without prior referrals, and case-finding, or seeking out need. Attention is drawn to the wide variety of activity involved. This chapter will also describe and examine the interventions made by the project nurse, and describe his experience and interactions with the residents and others he met during the study. In Chapter 6, reactive district nursing intervention, that is, intervention in response to referral, will be examined. At the heart of the study's analysis, evaluation and recommendations will be the comparison and implications for nursing practice of these two forms of district nursing intervention.

Of particular importance to readers is that this chapter will exemplify how the project nurse, a qualified district nurse but one who had never before worked with hostel residents, was able to record phenomena, interventions and interactions in a fast-moving, unstructured situation. The techniques he used, it is strongly suggested, are relevant and may be useful to any professional seeking to work effectively in a similar area. The chapter will also show how the project nurse created structures and developed systems to maximize his nursing influence and his recording potential.

Finally, this chapter will highlight the physical and psychiatric morbidity discovered during the assessments and interventions, as well as providing with a discussion of some of the positive adaptations made by the men.

Project nurse's diary

The project nurse was introduced to the hostel staff by the author during the first week of his employment on the study. From that time on, he kept an incident diary in which he recorded events and interactions. He recorded single-sentence comments – ideas, feelings and observations that occurred to him as he proceeded to set up his modes of operation. At a later time, when he returned to the study office, he used these comments reflectively to inform his practice.

For example, the project nurse recorded occasions when staff and residents described to him the problems suffered by residents who had not approached him. This information assisted the project nurse in devising strategies for contacting these and other residents by letter, and by varying the times of his attendance.

Nursing assessment

As well as the incident diary, the project nurse administered the interview containing the questionnaire and the validated tools (see Appendix I). The responses gained from this part of the study produced the results that were discussed in Chapter 4, with its concentration on a description of the samples in the Main Study and Comparison Hostels attained by using a statistical analysis of the data.

In the Main Study Hostel, the project nurse also used the interview, containing the questionnaire and the validated tools, as the first part of an individual nursing assessment for each resident interviewed. As the interview with each resident progressed, the project nurse noted in his incident diary any health needs that emerged from the resident's responses.

Having completed the first two parts of the data collection, the project nurse then proceeded to the third section, which comprised the structured questionnaire of 10 questions 'Brief Objective Measures for the Determination of Mental Status in the Elderly' (Khan et al 1960). This was administered to residents of 60 years and over. The assessment continued with a semi-structured interview using as a framework Roper et al's (1990) Activities of Daily Living. As will be seen in Appendix I, each activity is followed by a series of prompts.

At the end of this nursing assessment, in order to summarize and focus the process, the resident was asked specifically what problems he had and what he would like done for him.

Finally, the project nurse considered the question 'Does this resident need nursing and/or medical attention?' If the answer was 'No' – that is, the resident did not ask for help and the project nurse had not discovered any need at that time – the resident was thanked and the interview concluded. In all cases, the project nurse emphasized to the resident that he was free to come and visit again at any time. If, however, the answer was 'Yes', the project nurse continued the interview (see Appendix I and Chapter 3) to the section on 'Planning for Intervention and Intervention'.

Themes from the reflective tool

The purpose of the reflective tool (see Appendix I) was to help the project nurse to plan any necessary intervention following his assessment based upon Roy's adaptation theory and model (Roy 1980, Aggleton and Chalmers 1986). The tool comprised questions for the project nurse to consider. These focused on the resident's condition and experience under each of Roy's (1980) four adaptive modes: physiological, self-concept, role function and interdependency. Roy's theory recognizes that an individual's ability to adapt to external forces (stimuli) is affected by factors described in the four adaptive modes.

From the literature, particularly the five projects examined in detail in Chapter 2, the author had discovered that the care of homeless people had not only been concerned with identifying morbidity and treating the related problems or referring them to other agencies: factors such as the individual's perception of his state of health and his motivation were also important. The reflective tool attempted to elicit the individual's perception of his condition and the difficulties he encountered.

The use of this reflective tool was intended to assist the project nurse in gaining a greater insight into the individual residents' needs and experience. Table 5.1 shows that nine main themes emerged from the process of its use and the analysis of the results.

During the study, health and other professionals commented to the project nurse on the poor environment of the Main Study Hostel and how they felt that this must influence the residents' motivation to keep healthy or seek help. This environmental factor was found to be relevant in nine cases, in which residents actually expressed to the project nurse that the hostel had a negative influence on them (theme A). This number, however, represents only those who made this problem explicit.

More specifically, the residents also remarked how difficult it was to keep themselves and their clothes clean and, for some, how the absence of a working lift made it difficult for them to move around the hostel.

Table 5.1: Themes from the reflective tool.

Theme		Number of occurences recorded
Theme A	Resident affected by poor hostel facilities	9
Theme B	1. Peer pressure – difficulty in giving up alcohol	12
	2. Peer pressure – difficulty in giving up drugs	5
Theme C	Infestation	3
Theme D	Resident aware of health problem but not consulting the GP	9
Theme E	Resident not aware of health problem	13
Theme F	Sleeping difficulties	3
Theme G	Family relationship problems	20
Theme H	Resident feels rejected by family	12
Theme I	Resident has difficulty communicating with other residents	7

Distance from the toilets was also a problem for some of the frailer men. In addition, three men complained of having difficulty sleeping (theme F), the noisy hostel environment being stated as a contributing factor.

Theme B depicts a number of men (17) who expressed to the project nurse that they wanted to stop or control their excessive drug or alcohol use, but felt that the social environment was a barrier to their being able to address their problem. Conversely, the project nurse also found that many of the men did not see their use of drugs or alcohol as a problem.

Although only three men complained to the project nurse of infestation (theme C) the hostel staff and other health professionals recognized infestation, particularly body lice, as an ongoing problem. The lack of laundry facilities and general low standards of hygiene were also viewed as contributory factors. The project nurse became involved in treating infested residents, particularly when individuals considered their condition to be a barrier to seeking mainstream health care.

The project nurse also found nine men who were aware of some of health-related problems but did not seek help from their general practitioner (GP) (theme D). Some of these men attended their GP on a regular basis for prescriptions and sickness certificates but did not engage in a dialogue regarding other problems. A number of the men described to the project nurse how they did not think that it would make much difference to them if they addressed these problems, and they were not particularly worried. Others were concerned but appeared to feel hopeless about their condition, especially if they had alcohol abuse problems.

The project nurse also discovered that, following his nursing assessment and the identification of health needs, 13 of the residents were unaware of any health problems (theme E). This number represents approximately a fifth of the residents who received intervention.

The importance of this factor became apparent during the intervention stage. The project nurse noted how some residents did respond to his referral to a health professional after the resident had approached the project nurse (expressed need). The project nurse also compared the responses of some residents whose referrals emanated from his nursing assessment alone (unexpressed need). This will be discussed further in Chapter 10.

Attention is drawn to the number of men (20 in theme G) who expressed to the project nurse that family relationship problems had been a significant factor in their being in the hostel, and that this had also affected their health and motivation. Several explained to the project nurse how they tended 'not to bother' with their health since they had become estranged from and/or rejected by their families (theme H).

Seven men (theme I) expressed to the project nurse how they had difficulty interacting with other residents. This made life difficult for them as the residents all lived so closely together, and for many the friendship of other residents was the only opportunity available to interact with other people. This isolation will be discussed in Chapter 8.

At the conclusion of the study, the project nurse was asked whether he had found the tool useful as an aid to planning intervention. He stated that, in relation to his practical nursing intervention, he had in most cases already decided during the assessment what nursing intervention would be required. However, the tool had the beneficial effect of helping him to appreciate the complexity of the men's experience and of the interlinking of physical signs, such as excessive alcohol use, with other factors such as difficulty in communicating and the experience of feelings of rejection.

It was only by considering both the presenting nursing needs together with these underlying factors, which affected the individual's adaptation to help and his ability to respond, that the project nurse was able to proceed to the intervention stage. The adaptation processes of the men will be discussed in detail in Chapter 8. It is important to emphasize that the study was attempting not only to identify physical and psychiatric morbidity and make referrals, but also to engage the project nurse in an involvement with the men at a more complex level. The reflective tool assisted in this process.

Paradigms

From the beginning of the study, the project nurse collected paradigms, which demonstrated the experiences he encountered, the themes that were recognized and the perceptual shifts in the project nurse's understanding of these experiences. These paradigms will be used in this and subsequent chapters to elucidate phenomena and to complement statistical data, especially where one man's story summarizes the experience of many. Another important feature of the paradigms is in giving the reader an insight into the sample subjects' lives, their experience of their physical and social environment, and their interaction with the project nurse.

Assessments and interventions

It will be seen in Table 5.2 that most of the encounters with the project nurse took place as a result of contact in the communal areas of the hostel during normal office hours. It was decided to use two other methods of recruiting – written invitation and out-of-hours sessions – to discover whether this varied approach would assist recruitment to the study. The letter, followed by a visit from the project nurse to the resident's room, proved useful. Out-of-hours recruiting was less fruitful, but the project nurse considered it to be useful as he was able to contact some men who were not available at other times.

Just over half of the assessments and interventions undertaken by the project nurse were accomplished in the first 4 weeks of the study. It is also interesting to note that in the first few weeks, most of the men assessed needed intervention.

The project nurse found that news of his presence quickly brought some men to his door. After the first letter, the number of men assessed increased, but the need for intervention decreased, suggesting that many men were aware of their current needs, felt that they did not need care but were willing to take part in the study. The second and third letters produced a slight increase in uptake so that 106 men out of the total population of 168 took part in the study. Thirty-two other men were approached but refused to take part. Eight men approached the project nurse for help and received intervention, but they refused to take part in the study. After 11 weeks of systematic and varied recruiting practices, 22 men (13% of the total population) had not been seen at all by the project nurse.

Table 5.2: Patterns of recruiting by the project nurse

		Number of residents recruited
A	Approaches to residents and opportunistic encounters in communal areas in the hostel	60
B	Letters sent to residents seeking interview floor by floor, followed by a visit to the resident's room if required	34
C	Evening and early morning shift by the project nurse	12

Profile of the men who received intervention

The profile below highlights the comparisons and contrasts between the group of men who received intervention and those who did not. Its purpose is to gain further insight into the groups and into any implications for practice.

Age versus receipt of intervention

A significant difference was found between the residents who received intervention and those who did not (Table 5.3). Ten out of the 13 residents who were aged 25 years or less received intervention. The project nurse found that many of the younger men were not altogether satisfied with his help and may, therefore, have been more motivated to change their circumstances. The project nurse also found that many of them had drug and alcohol misuse problems, and four men scored over 10 on the Hospital Anxiety and Depression (HAD) Scale for depression, suggesting that they may have been suffering from biogenic depression.

Another reason for the higher number of younger men needing intervention may have been that they were leading a more unhealthy, chaotic lifestyle and were more unsettled than the older residents. The project nurse's detailed notes recorded the physical and psychological distress displayed by some of the residents, particularly young men. A more in-depth analysis of these observations will take place in Chapter 8, a discussion of the different subgroups of residents being found in Chapter 9.

Table 5.3: Residents' ages compared with intervention and non-interventions.

	Age				
	25 and under	26–50 years	51–70 years	71+ years	Total
Interventions	10	18	32	6	66
Non-interventions	3	41	53	5	102
Total	13	59	85	11	168

Chi-squared test, p = <0.001.

Length of stay in the Main Study Hostel versus receipt of intervention

Table 5.4 shows that more than half of the men receiving intervention had been staying in the hostel for under a year, whereas most of those who did not receive intervention had been there between 1 and 5 years. The Chi-square test showed this to be significant difference. It was apparent to the project nurse, from the HAD Scale scores and from his assessments, that some men might have become resident as a result of psychiatric and physical morbidity, particularly depression and alcohol use. The Main Study Hostel was also considered to be a place of last resort where men who had been banned from other hostels came. This will be discussed in Chapter 9.

Visits to accident and emergency

Also statistically significant was the fact that the group of men who received intervention had visited the accident and emergency (A and E) department almost twice as often as those who did not receive intervention (Table 5.5). This may be connected with the high

Table 5.4: Residents' length of stay compared with intervention and non-interventions.

	Length of stay			
	under 1 year	1–5 years	6+ years	Total
Interventions	32	14	12	58
Non-interventions	26	56	18	100
Total	58	70	30	158

Chi-squared test, p = <0.001.

Table 5.5: Visits by residents to A&E compared with intervention and non-interventions.

	Visits to A&E in the last 2 years				
	None	Once	Twice	More than 2	Total
Interventions	18	11	5	22	56
Non-interventions	18	7	2	2	29
Total	36	18	7	24	85

Chi-squared test, p = <0.001.

level of alcohol use problems. Sixteen out of the 22 men who received intervention and had been to A and E more than twice scored in the highest category of the impact of alcohol use.

It is interesting to note that 18 men in each group had never attended A and E. This suggests that residents have different lifestyles and that it would be a mistake to form rigid stereotypes of such men.

Impact of alcohol

Two-thirds of the men who required intervention scored highly in the impact that alcohol (Table 5.6) had on their lives, the Chi-square test showing this to be significant. This was also reflected in the project nurse's experience during the assessments.

Residents' feelings of health

The Chi-square test demonstrated a significant relationship between intervention and those men who said they felt unwell (Table 5.7). As

Table 5.6: Impact of residents' alcohol use on lifestyle compared with intervention and non-interventions.

	Impact of alcohol events					
	Doesn't drink	No events	Some events	Number of events	Considerable events	Total
Interventions	10	0	9	11	29	59
Non-interventions	6	3	6	6	8	29
Total	16	3	15	17	37	88

Chi-squared test, p = <0.001.

Table 5.7: Residents' feeling of health compared with intervention and non-interventions.

	Felt well	Felt unwell/ill	Total
Interventions	26	32	58
Non-interventions	23	6	29
Total	49	38	87

Chi-squared test, $p = <0.001$.

mentioned in Chapter 4, the question 'How do you feel?' proved very useful in this study as residents appeared to answer truthfully – if they felt well they said so. This result, therefore, did not support the statements made by some health professionals to the author and project nurse, that they would expect the men to say that they were unwell in order to receive attention.

Conclusion

Although no statistically significant differences were discovered between the group of men who received intervention and those who did not, the group of men under 25 years of age figured highly in the intervention group, as did men who had been in the hostel less than a year. Those who received intervention tended to visit the A and E department more frequently, and half of the intervention group scored in the highest category for the impact of alcohol use. The practice implications of identifying young and new residents will be discussed further in Chapter 10.

Project nurse's interactions and interventions

The remainder of the chapter is an exposition of the interactions, interventions and discoveries made by the project nurse. The themes were created from the reflective analysis tool described above, the incident diary and the nursing assessment, and are listed below. A more detailed explanation of individual themes and interventions follows, these being exemplified by paradigms.

List of themes

Group theme: service themes

- Service failing to meet resident's needs
- Resident in regular contact with health or social service
- Referral from hostel staff.

Group theme: nursing action themes

- Project nurse gains respect from resident(s) as a result of previous intervention
- Referral to hostel team
- Project nurse uses professional judgement to limit the extent of intervention
- Project nurse intervention recognized as being important by the resident.

Group theme: positive adaptation themes

- Resident a 'regular customer' of the project nurse
- Resident adaptation to the intervention or advice of the project nurse
- Resident seeking assistance with an alcohol misuse problem
- Resident seeking assistance with a drug misuse problem
- Resident refers another resident to the project nurse
- Resident caring for another resident
- Resident seeking assistance to find alternative accommodation.

Group theme: negative adaptation themes

- Access to GP service limited:
  – distance to GP too far
  – resident reluctant to visit GP
  – resident not registered with a GP
- Resident avoiding responsibility by deferring to the project nurse
- Resident regularly visits GP but does not discuss health problems
- Resident fails to keep an appointment made for him by the project nurse
- Resident refuses to take part in the study
- Resident refuses to complete the assessment
- Resident suspicious of the project nurse
- Resident suspicious of aggressive behaviour.

Group theme: morbidity

- Resident infested
- Resident has a history of mental illness
- Resident has signs of physical illness
- Resident's Barthel score satisfactory but resident obviously physically compromised.

Service themes

Eighty-six per cent (137) of the men in the Main Study Hostel were registered with a GP, and the majority of those seen by the project nurse had seen their GP within the past 3 months. The project nurse quickly discovered that many of the men had expressed their health and nursing needs to hostel and other professionals, and/or that these professionals were aware that they needed help. Seventeen men were receiving a service from health and/or social services. Some men stated that the services they were receiving did not meet their needs.

As soon as he began the study, the project nurse was approached by and received 10 referrals from the hostel staff, who were worried about the condition of the men. The deficit demonstrated was that there was a knowledge of some men's conditions, but that a gap existed between the knowledge and action. An example of a referral from hostel staff is described in this paradigm (written in the project nurse's words).

> J.B. is a 78-year-old man who has stayed in the hostel for 58 years. Most of his working life was spent at sea on merchant and cruise ships. Because of this, he never established a settled home. During this time, he stayed at the Main Study Hostel between jobs. It was therefore a natural progression for him to take up full-time residence after retiring.
>
> He was referred to me by the hostel staff as he had been complaining of pain in his right groin. On examination, I found that he had a right inguinal hernia. He also complained of lower back pain. Further examination revealed that he was also infested with scabies.
>
> I arranged a GP appointment and treated the scabies with Quellada. As he was rather frail, I decided to accompany him to the appointment. On arriving at the health centre, I discovered that he was not registered with the GP with whom he had stated he was registered. However, the GP agreed to take him on. As a result of attending the GP, he now receives regular prescriptions for oral analgesia and an analgesic cream, and was referred for surgery for his inguinal hernia.

It may be seen how the project nurse not only assessed this resident's needs and made provisional diagnoses, but also bridged gaps for the hostel staff, who knew that the resident needed help but did not know what to do. The project nurse made links between the hostel and the services by referring the resident and then preparing him for his appointment by disinfesting him and accompanying him to the GP.

Referrals from other residents

Some men who visited the project nurse were recommended by other residents, five men, who were worried about their five neighbours, directly approaching him and referring residents to him. This was a useful contact as some of these men were in a poor state of health. The following paradigm illustrates one man's experience.

> J.L. is a 53-year-old man with alcohol-related problems who suffers from epilepsy. My first encounter with him was as a result of a referral from another resident, who informed me that J.L. had been having fits during the night. When I went to see him, he was obviously in a post-ictal state. He was unable to recognize his friend or respond to verbal commands. When I approached the staff, I was informed that they were aware that he had been having convulsions, but he had been responsive earlier in the morning. As a result, an ambulance was called and he was admitted to hospital. A search of his room revealed that he had several empty bottles of anticonvulsants but no current prescription.

> After his discharge from hospital, I approached him on a few occasions in an attempt to assess him properly. However, he was not prepared to take part in the assessment.

The project nurse found many examples of friendship and neighbourliness among the men, as well as isolation and loneliness. The above paradigm is a demonstration of a resident trying to get help for his friend. The project nurse also found in this case, and in others, difficulty in assisting some men who had been referred by someone else; that is, the uptake of help appeared to be better when the individual recognized and expressed a need himself.

Morbidity

The project nurse found, as expected from the literature, a large number of men with a great variety of illnesses and histories of treatment. One group who became particularly important to this study were those, mainly old, men who were physically surviving in the hostel but only just. Fourteen men scored highly on the Barthel Index for physical function but on assessment were found to be far from well. For example, as assessed by the Barthel Index, some could climb the stairs and go to the toilet, but observation by the project nurse showed that this took them 15 or 20 minutes. In the previous chapter, it was noted that this was a reflection on the Main Study Hostel's facilities – no downstairs toilets and no lifts – and that the Barthel score can be as much an indication of the ability of a building to support disabled people as it is an image of the individual.

The study also found that many of the men living 'on the edge' in this manner would, when they became ill, rapidly deteriorate and become completely disabled within a matter of days. One man was observed to deteriorate from a situation of reasonable function and self-care to one of complete debility in just 3 days.

Negative adaptations by residents

Some residents were openly hostile to the project nurse, while others were reluctant to see their GP or, if they did visit, did not discuss their problems in any detail. Another group of men had a tendency to place the responsibility for their expressed problems entirely onto the project nurse, with little or no contribution from themselves: 'You must do something about this' was a typical directive. These men proved difficult to help as the project nurse was reliant on the co-operation of the men to take up the referrals, advocacies and advice he offered.

Table 5.8 lists some of these 'negative adaptations' and how often the project nurse encountered and recorded them as he made the nursing assessments and engaged the men in conversation. These responses demonstrate that it was not just a question of the project nurse discovering morbidity and making an appropriate intervention. As described earlier, the attitude of the individual was important, as was his previous experience of the health services.

Table 5.8: Negative adaptations

Negative adaptation	Number of residents
Service access limited because:	
• too far from GP	15
• resident reluctant to see GP	27
• resident not registered with GP	14
Resident avoiding responsibility by passing it to the project nurse	14
Regular visits to GP without discussing all health problems	5
Resident failed to keep appointment made by the project nurse	17
Resident suspicious of project nurse	21

Table 5.9: Treatments

Treatment	Number of residents
Dressing wound	13
Disinfestation/bathing	10
Bathing prior to appointment	2
First aid to resident with seizure	1
First aid to resident with injury	2
Cutting nails	2
Pressure area care	1
Removal of sutures	3

Interventions

Treatment administered by the project nurse

One of the main skills associated with district nursing is the ability to treat people in a variety of situations, particularly in terms of the care of their skin and wounds (Table 5.9). In this study, treatment was provided by the project nurse when it could not be deferred because the need was immediate.

Another rationale for immediate treatment was demonstrated by the number of men who were disinfested. The project nurse acted as a bridge between the hostel and the health services by getting residents 'fit to be seen'. This action was not necessarily a value judgement on the part of the project nurse, as the men would often not go to see their GP because of shame and embarrassment.

The following paradigm exemplifies the project nurse treating a resident. It demonstrates how the ability to treat a man with an immediate practical remedy was a beneficial tool for the project nurse. It gave an entry into the patient's life, particularly as he and many others either were not very articulate or were suspicious of the service.

R.P. was a 63-year-old man, referred to me by hostel staff. He was unkempt and dirty. On examination, I found his legs to be badly excoriated due to scratching. A similar rash was found on his arms, shoulders and back. The appearance and widespread nature of the rash indicated that it was caused by scabies. After assisting R.P. to bath, apply Quellada lotion and find him some clean clothing, I was able to assess him properly as he was in a much better frame of mind and felt better.

Assessment of R.P. revealed two other problems. He complained of pain in his left leg. This appeared to come from the site of a fracture that had required internal fixation. The other problem was bilateral cataract. He had attended an optician in 1991 and had been informed of this problem. Further questioning revealed that he had not consulted for over 6 years. I persuaded R.P. that both these matters were important enough to warrant visiting his GP, and arranged the appointment for him.

As a result of attending this appointment, R.P. received analgesia and was referred to Glasgow Royal Infirmary for ophthalmic assessment. Subsequently, he arranged and attended a second GP appointment, and is being admitted for ophthalmic surgery.

The paradigm above highlights the difficulty that some hostel-dwellers had in accessing the available services. This problem arose not as a result of any barriers put up by the service but from the individual's inability to recognize (a) that he had a problem, (b) that treatment was available, and (c) that gaining access to this treatment generally required attendance at a GP.

The project nurse also found that some men came to him for treatment for one complaint, as a result of which he gained an insight into other areas of the patient's life. The following paradigm illustrates this point.

B.W. is a 30-year-old with a drinking problem who suffers from epilepsy. My first encounter with him came as a result of being called to attend him while he was having a grand mal seizure in the TV room.

He approached me 2 weeks later concerned about a hand laceration that he thought might be infected. On examination, this was found not to be the case. During the assessment, he told me that he had run out of antiepileptic medication but had a GP appointment in 2 weeks. I advised him that as his epilepsy was clearly poorly controlled, he should attend his GP sooner.

The project nurse often found that men presented to him overtly worried about one thing but demonstrating general underlying anxiety and distress, for which the project nurse felt he could do very little. Thus, whereas the ability to treat was a good entry into a resident's problems, it did not necessarily make solving them any easier.

Referrals by the project nurse

Table 5.10 shows the range of referrals made by the project nurse. During the time of the study, the community psychiatric nursing (CPN) hostel team also commenced its service in Glasgow. A working

Table 5.10: Referrals

	Number of residents
Registered resident with GP	8
Psychiatric problem to GP	30
Physical problem to GP	30
To GP for alcohol rehabilitation	7
Ambulance to A&E	1
CPN	32
District nurse	6
Social work team	3
Hostel social work team	7
To GP for substance abuse	1
Clinical Psychologist	1

relationship was made between the project nurse and the CPN. This was an important point gleaned from the study as it demonstrated the usefulness of referral networks, that is, the importance of the referrer, in this case the project nurse, establishing a relationship with the referees, here the CPN hostel team. The subsequent actions of the practitioners who received referrals will be discussed in Chapter 6.

It is important to emphasize here that the project nurse was able to assess a large number of residents to a level such that he could make written referrals to other agencies (see Appendix II).

The number of referrals made for physical problems should be highlighted here. Emphasis has been laid in the literature and by policy-makers on the psychiatric needs of the homeless (the only specialist nursing team for the homeless in Glasgow being a psychiatric team). The present study also discovered much psychiatric illness, but it also found a large physical need. The project nurse, a district nurse acting as a generalist, was able to respond to both physical and psychiatric need. The benefits of the district nurse as a generalist will be discussed in Chapter 10.

Mental health referrals

The referrals for psychiatric care were mainly associated with a high depression score on the HAD Scale. The 22 men who scored 10 or over (see Chapter 4), signifying that they might be suffering from biogenic depression, were referred to their GP and to the CPN. Men who scored highly for anxiety were not referred for that alone, as anxiety by itself is not a psychiatric condition. However, if they were being referred to the GP or district nurse for another reason, the high anxiety score was included in the referral.

At this point, it is relevant to state that although many of the men did not co-operate with the study, the project nurse considered that many were still in need. This became particularly apparent when dealing with residents with psychotic illnesses. The project nurse discovered that even where proper assessment and referral was possible and appropriate referrals were made, often with personal contact with and agreement on the part of health professionals, it was still either very difficult or impossible to provide a service that met the resident's needs. To demonstrate this lack of progress and ability to deliver a service, the following paradigm describes two residents

I.K. was a 70-year-old man about whom the staff had become concerned as a result of changes in his behaviour. He was a long-term resident and therefore well known to the staff. Over the course of a few weeks, he became forgetful and was expressing paranoid ideas. At the time I became involved, he was already being visited by a CPN.

On our first meeting, I.K. expressed ideas that may or may not have been viewed as paranoid. He complained of harassment from the 'management', who would wake him up at night. He was afraid of being locked up in a dungeon that he said was in the basement. He also stated that the manager had told him to leave the hostel. His statements were inconsistent with the concern shown by the staff in general, and the manager in particular, about his welfare.

The CPN involved arranged a GP visit. His GP found him to be hypertensive, but I.K. refused treatment. When I contacted the GP, he told me that he found no sign of paranoia. He went on to say, however, that for a Jewish man to be living in the Great Eastern Hotel there must be some psychological disturbance present. He further stated that a crisis situation would have to develop before he could take any further action.

On the second occasion that I talked with I.K., I found him to be very guarded in what he said. Prior to this meeting, the manager had told me that I.K. had torn up his pension book, stating that someone was going to take it off him. It was clear during our meeting that he did not trust me, and he gave little away.

On the third meeting (the formal assessment), he was again expressing paranoid ideas. He stated that people from a block of flats opposite were threatening him. He made a reference to a knife but did not expand on this. During this meeting, it was apparent that he was experiencing auditory hallucinations.

As a result of this assessment, I wrote to his GP reaffirming my belief that I.K. was suffering from a psychiatric disorder. I also referred him to the Hostel Care Team (Social Work Department) for assessment as I felt that he would benefit from regular contact with someone from outside the hostel.

I.K. continued in this indeterminate state throughout the period of the study. No one was actively preventing him gaining help, but no progress was made despite collaborative efforts.

V.F. is a 57-year-old man. He is usually observed standing next to the drinks machine talking to it, in the corridor between the reception area and the dining room, surrounded by various hold-alls and carrier bags containing all his worldly possessions. While standing there, he appears to respond to auditory hallucinations and has heated conversations using a variety of voices. Despite his obvious psychiatric problems, he appears to be able to communicate in an appropriate manner when required to do so.

I approached him on three occasions for an interview, but he politely declined on each occasion. As his chosen territory was just outside the office I used for interviews, I made a point of exchanging pleasantries with him whenever I passed. I decided to refer him to the CPN service despite not having completed an assessment.

It appears that he will not be followed up because he failed to exhibit psychotic behaviour during the interview with the CPN. This is surprising in view of the considerable anecdotal evidence from myself and the hostel staff regarding his unusual behaviour. While I accept that it would be inappropriate to force treatment on this individual, I do feel that he should have been retained as a current case for follow-up and monitoring.

V.F. demonstrated another problem in that even if it had been possible to treat his psychosis, one would still have been left with a man who had very little social context, companionship or meaningful lifestyle. He still spends his days walking purposefully round Glasgow or talking to the drinks machine. Always he carries his heavy plastic bags. He does not speak to anyone, and has no friends. The author and project nurse discovered no answer to this dilemma.

Non-compliant residents

Many of the residents referred for help appeared to be in an agitated state, wanting help but not necessarily responding to the project nurse's referrals. They seemed tortured and overwhelmed by their life and experience. P.D. was an example of this.

P.D. was a 25-year-old man who had been living in homeless accommodation since his late teens. He had a number of physical and psychological problems. He complained specifically of dyspnoea, chest pains, back pains, leg pains and depression. He was also worried about his obesity and alcoholism. He scored highly on both the HAD Scales. His main reason for approaching me was to get a 'physical-check up' as he was about to commence a work experience programme.

As a result of the assessment, I advised P.D. that I thought that he would benefit from attending his GP and talking with a CPN. Initially, he agreed to me referring him to both. Two days later, however, he came back to me and said that he did not wish to see either the GP or the CPN.

On enquiring as to the reason for the change of mind, he told me that he did not think that he had a mental health problem. After a period of negotiation, I persuaded him to allow me to refer him to his GP for the physical problems. This involved writing the referral letter in his presence and allowing him to approve it. I then made the GP appointment for him.

When I next saw him, a few weeks later, he told me that he had not attended the appointment. I advised him to make another appointment with the GP. He left the hostel soon after this meeting.

This resident, as with many others, could be labelled 'non-compliant'. The author and project nurse recognized that a study involving referrals will include subjects who do not comply. This, and other issues associated with negative adaptations or responses by residents to the project nurse's interventions, will be discussed in Chapters 8 and 10.

Advocacy

Advocacy was, in terms of the study, defined as actions taken by the project nurse that assisted a resident by word, letter or deed but that were not treatments or referrals. Tables 5.11 and 5.12 demonstrate the variety of acts of advocacy performed by the project nurse. The main activity lay in arranging appointments for residents. Also important to the residents was that the project nurse made supportive communications to colleagues in other agencies, rather like the historical 'letters of reference' for travellers. This activity acted as a guarantee to the agency that the need was genuine, and was seen as a tangible expression of confidence and respect for the resident.

Similarly, accompanying men to appointments had a profound and positive effect on the individuals, particularly where the resident was elderly and/or frail and had communication difficulties. Although only

Table 5.11: Advocacies

Act of advocacy	Number of residents
Supporting telephone call to social security	2
Supporting telephone call to GP	9
Supporting telephone call to social worker	4
Accompanying resident to appointment	6
Approach to hostel management	3
Supporting telephone call to community psychiatric nurse	4
Assisting resident to complete form	3
Arranging an appointment	5
Supporting telephone call to consultant	3
Supporting telephone call to Health Board (GP registration)	3
Supporting telephone call to A&E department or outpatient clinic	2
Supporting letter to GP	1
Supporting telephone call to alcohol unit	3
Supporting letter to the Department of Social Security	1
Ordering repeat prescription for resident	1
Supporting letter to A&E	1

Table 5.12: Examples of acts by project nurse to support residents (22 in total)

Date	Activity
15.9.92	Accompanied JB to Bridgeton Health Centre for appointment with his GP
5.11.92	Wrote letter of support to Social Security
2.12.92	Phone Bridgeton Health Centre for repeat prescription for JB
3.12.92	Picked up prescription from Health Centre for JB
3.12.92	Took AS Glasgow Royal Infirmary A&E department
4. 2.93	Accompanied to JM to GRI A&E department stayed 4 hours

three men were helped to fill in forms, part of the general activity of the project nurse in his interactions with the men was to help them to understand the working practices and machinery of the health and other services.

Advice

During the time of the study, the project nurse was asked many questions by residents, mostly by those participating in the study but also by other men in the hostel. His presence created a focus, and he was able to provide relevant information both during the course of the interviews and to men who approached him in the hostel (Table 5.13). It is difficult to measure the success of advice-giving in these circumstances,

Table 5.13: Advice given to residents

Advice	Number of residents
To register with GP	12
To make appointment with GP	34
To attend social work	22
To attend housing	3
To attend optician	1
To accept nursing treatment	4
To attend A&E department at Glasgow Royal Infirmary	3

but from the variety of questions received, it certainly seemed to be beneficial to the residents concerned that the project nurse had the health and welfare knowledge of a district nurse.

Activity in the hostel not generated by the project nurse

During the time of the study, the CPN from the hostel team visited twice a week, as did the social work hostel care team, seeing several residents. A district nurse visited one resident monthly. Table 5.14 demonstrates the activity in the hostel generated by health and other professionals. All of these professionals were acting in response to a referral from hostel staff and, in a few cases, to self-referral. No interactions took place as a result of regular monitoring visits. The opportunities that this activity creates for the regular assessment and monitoring by health professionals of residents in hostels and similar places of need will be discussed in Chapter 10.

Table 5.14: Examples of activity of other health professionals within the Main Study Hostel during the study not initiated by the project nurse (30 incidents in total)

Date	Activity
12. 8.92	CPN visits I.K.
26. 8.92	CPN visits I.K.
27. 8.92	GP visits I.K.
24. 9.92	CPN visits three residents
9.10.92	R.G. admitted to Glasgow Royal Infirmary (lung cancer)
17.10.92	Ambulance called by one of the residents for F.M. (head injury)
8.12.92	GP called out to A.L.
9.12.92	Community mental handicap nurse visits S.B.
10.12.92	CPN visits residents

Work with the tuberculosis screening unit

While the author and project nurse were involved in the fieldwork, they were asked to assist the Greater Glasgow Health Board Screening Unit to recruit as many residents as possible to attend for a chest X-ray. The men were offered meal vouchers and transport if required. The project nurse helped hostel staff to disseminate information about the screening.

Over 3 days, 100 men were screened, which was reported to be a large improvement on previous years. Ten men were found to have an abnormal X-ray. Two were found to have malignancies, two emphysema and six tuberculosis. These six were referred to hospital physicians. They kept their appointments and were treated. However, it is not known by the author and the project nurse whether these men continued to comply in the long term.

For ethical reasons the Screening Unit and the study did not exchange precise patient details. This interlude was interesting for two main reasons. First, the Screening Unit informed the author that six cases was a very high incidence of tuberculosis, even taking into account recent increases. In the normal population, the incidence had been so low that a figure was not given. The unit was not altogether surprised at this high incidence in the hostel, which was the reason why regular screening was offered to hostel residents. Second, the compliance rate for follow-up appointments and treatments was very high. This may reflect the seriousness in which the term 'TB' is held by residents.

Positive adaptations

This chapter has attempted to display the variety and complexity of the project nurse's interventions and interactions with the residents and the hostel and health professionals. He encountered a number of difficulties, both in terms of interpersonal communication and in making appropriate responses to need. As has been described, he found that many men did not take up the appointments that had been made for them. However, the project nurse found that many men did make adaptations and not only kept appointments, but also kept in touch with him or involved other residents.

Attention is drawn to the six men shown in Table 5.15 who approached the project nurse because they were looking after other residents, and the five referrals from residents. Although low in percentage terms, these 11 men demonstrate that positive interactions with others are possible even in the most inhospitable venues. The project nurse also noticed the number of men who had not 'given up'

Table 5.15: Positive adaptation themes

	Number of residents
'Regular customers' (residents who visited the project nurse on a regular basis)	10
Resident requesting assistance with an alcohol problem	8
Resident requesting assistance with a drug problem	3
Referrals from other residents	5
Resident looking after other residents	6
Resident requesting assistance to find alternative accommodation	17

but were actively seeking alternative accommodation, some of whom had been looking for a considerable period of time. Seventeen of these men approached him for assistance to find housing.

Summary and conclusion

The previous chapter provided an exposition and discussion of the statistical data emanating from the assessment questionnaire and validated tools. Comparisons were made between the Main Study Hostel and another hostel. The present chapter describes how the project nurse gathered the mainly qualitative data, made nursing assessments and demonstrated the variety and complexity of his interventions and interactions with the residents and other professionals. The procedure proved successful and comprehensive.

Most of the assessments and interventions were carried out during the first 4 weeks of the fieldwork in the Main Study Hostel. As expected, considerable physical and psychiatric morbidity was discovered. A significant number of young men required intervention, as did many who had been in the hostel for a year or less. Most of the men had seen their GP recently, but many of them had not discussed their problems.

The uptake of the project nurse's interventions appeared to be connected to whether the individual had identified the problem for himself. Some of the men did not take up appointments made for them even though they still displayed need. Treatments by the project nurse provided a good entry into a resident's life as they were practical and appreciated, providing a bridge between the hostel and the health services.

Written referrals were made, but it was also important for the project nurse to create communication and referral networks with health professionals. A large number of advocacy acts were undertaken. The most important features of these acts were to recommend the individual to other professionals and to raise the man's confidence and feeling of worth. These acts appeared to be at least as important to the men as were treatments and referrals.

The project nurse recorded activity in the hostel by other health professionals, generated not by the study but in response to specific requests. This activity may present an opportunity for more strategic assessment and monitoring of hostels and will be discussed in Chapter 10.

Chapter 6
Evaluation of the health professionals' responses

The previous chapter examined the data collected by the project nurse as he assessed the residents and made interventions. This chapter will explore first the referrals made to the general practitioners (GPs) and community psychiatric nurse (CPN). Second, the results of the referrals will be evaluated. The GPs' and CPN's general feelings and ideas regarding the provision of health care for homeless men will be presented.

Finally, a detailed exposition will be presented of the referrals made to the district nurses. These were important for the study as they demonstrated the role of the district nurse as a reactive specialist, that is, responding to a referral for a specific set of skills and activities. It will be seen that a marked difference was found between this role and the project nurse's role acting as a proactive generalist, that is, case-finding, assessing and referring.

Referrals and follow-up

All the medical and nursing staff received a written referral from the project nurse (see Appendix II). These were followed up 6–12 weeks later by the author, who approached all the medical and nursing health professionals within Glasgow who had received referrals. Each practitioner who agreed to be interviewed was seen in his or her own office. A semi-structured interview took place (see Appendix I). The interviews took between 15 and 30 minutes, depending on how many referrals the practitioner had received. The exception to this concerned the CPN, who had received 31 referrals; the author's interview with her took two and a half hours.

The GP

It will be seen in Table 6.1 that the project nurse sent referrals to 23 GPs regarding 51 residents. One GP was found not to exist (the resident had given a false name). One GP was based in Lanarkshire 20 miles away and had had no contact with the resident, thus declining to take part in the interview. Another GP was not interviewed because the resident had left the hostel and the area almost immediately after the assessment and referral by the project nurse. One other GP declined to take part in the interview. One resident named a GP trainee as his doctor, which suggests recent, previous contact. In this case, the author interviewed the resident's GP. A total of 18 GPs therefore completed the interviews and reported on the care of 41 residents.

GP responses to the evaluation questionnaire

Four GPs visited five residents in the Main Study Hostel (Table 6.2).

Table 6.1: List of referrals made to health professionals

GP ID	Health centre	Referrals		
		GP	DN	CPN
209	Bridgeton	4	1	2
202		3	2	
208		6	1	3
205		4	1	3
212		2		2
206		5		4
204		3		2
202		3		1
213		2		
207		1		
219	Anderson	1		1
215	Townhead	1	1	
216		1		1
217		1		
218		1		1
220	Glenbarr St	1		
221	Shettleston	1		1
222	Woodside	1		1
Subtotal (18 GPs interviewed)		41		
2 GPs refused interview		2		1
GP did not exist		1		1
GP interviewed		1		1
Residents not referred to GP		6		6
Total referrals		51	6	31

DN = district nurse; CPN = community psychiatric nurse.

Table 6.2: GPs responses to 'What did you do as a result of the nursing referral you received regarding this resident?'

Responses	Number	Responses	Number
Visited resident in hostel	5	Arranged psychiatrist	1
No action taken	19	Made appointment to see GP	5
Patient not registered	3	Referred to geriatrician	3
Patient moved away	1	Referred to surgeon	2
Saw another partner	1	Referred to physician	2
Patient told to change GP	2		
Patient saw locum	1	*Referred to:*	
Patient prescribed medication	12	Eventide accommodation	1
Prescribed anticonvulsant	2	Social work	1
Prescribed antidepressant	1	Drug user help	1
(HAD Scale normal)			
Prescribed stockings	2	Letter for Department of	
Sent away until sober	2	Social Security	1
Sent for X-ray	1		

Of these five visits, two were made within 2 days of referral and the other three within a period of a few weeks. Three visits were made in response to a number of factors, the project nurse's referral playing an important role. Other factors were requests from hostel staff, the resident and the CPN. No action was taken in 19 of the referrals, but this was not necessarily because the GP thought the referral inappropriate, as will be described in detail later.

Fourteen different interventions were described, the prescription of medication being the most frequent. It is interesting to note that only one resident was prescribed antidepressants, although his Hospital Anxiety and Depression (HAD) Scale score was found by the author to be within the normal range. Twelve men, who were registered with GPs, scored highly for depression on the HAD scale; all were referred to their GP. None of these men received medication or referral. The validity of the HAD Scale will be discussed in Chapters 7 and 9.

In response to the author's questions, a general impression was gained from all the health professionals that the help possible for this group was limited. In addition, one of the main causes of this difficulty was the residents' environment: 'Well, he would be expected to be depressed living there' or 'It's not surprising he's in poor physical shape'. The most frequently cited cause of difficulty in delivering health services to homeless men was the residents' poor motivation, which was recognized by the GPs in eight specific cases.

When asked 'How did you come to make your decisions (regarding the nursing referral)?', the GPs generally confined themselves to any specific morbidity of which the resident complained. In two cases, a significant psychiatric history was recognized immediately: one resident was hallucinating, and the other had paranoid delusions. Single cases of varicose veins, Parkinson's disease, inguinal hernia, myocardial infarction, nausea and vomiting and breathing difficulties were also cited as factors that prompted action. One resident had called the GP out at night, and another had been brought to the GP's surgery by the project nurse.

In six cases, however, GPs recognized the need for monitoring and supervision, and considered a nursing service to be useful for this purpose. Regular visits by residents and good motivation were regarded as key factors contributing to positive intervention by the GPs in eight cases. The GPs in these eight cases considered regular interaction to be an important feature as it promoted the relationship between doctor and patient. This factor will be discussed further in Chapter 8.

The GPs were asked whether they had any difficulty putting their plan into action. Eleven of the men did not turn up for their appointment. A few of these were seen at a later date, but the majority were not. From a service point of view, it may be seen that this attrition rate poses a problem to GPs. This was compounded when six other residents refused the treatment prescribed. One factor described by the GPs in relation to the residents who refused was that they were able to diagnose the residents' ailments, but the residents did not necessarily recognize that a problem was present: 'I could see he had a problem, but he did not see it at all' was how one GP expressed himself.

Connected with this observation was the fact that two GPs proposed that the remedies and activities suggested to individuals, for example attending an outpatient appointment, lay outside the residents' normal range of daily activities and responses. This will be discussed in Chapter 8 and the service implications in Chapter 10.

Five GPs visited their patients, three finding it easy to locate their patient. The author received some general comments from health professionals on how mobile and transient the hostel population was. The author and project nurse did not find this to be the case in most instances, and the GPs in these five cases stated that their patients who were hostel residents tended to remain in the area most of the time.

The GPs were asked 'What was your opinion of your patient's physical and mental state?' In their replies, it was discovered that 12 patients were in a poor physical state, although only three (a resident with Parkinson's disease, one with breathing difficulties and another with varicose veins and walking difficulties) showed decreased physical function using the Barthel Index. The other nine residents were considered to be frail and physically vulnerable (six residents because of their alcohol misuse and three because of their age).

Eleven residents were considered to be in a poor mental state, six of these also demonstrating a poor physical condition. Four were considered to be depressed. Of these four, one (whom, it was found, had scored within the normal range on the HAD scale) was given treatment for depression. Of the other two residents who were considered depressed, one had scored in the high range and the other in the intermediate range of the HAD scale.

These responses demonstrate the degree of physical and psychiatric morbidity found in this group. The GPs tended to recognize that there was a great deal of medical need in this group; their problem was how to meet it effectively.

When asked whether they thought the referrals from the project nurse had been useful, 20 GPs replied that they believed the referrals to be appropriate. In addition, six of the GPs (each of whom had received more than one referral) valued this kind of referral (from a nurse working in the field) as it provided a useful overview of the residents and updated their medical notes. Three GPs did not think that the referrals they received were appropriate. These three GPs had each received one referral; two did not feel that the resident's condition merited medical attention, and another stated that the resident was in prison.

In five cases, GPs discovered additional reasons not described by the project nurse's referral why their patients needed their attention. Three residents were found to have hypertension, one was arthritic, and another suffered from schizophrenia.

As has previously been stated, GPs tended not to investigate a resident's physical and psychiatric morbidity further than the presenting complaint, yet three men were found to have hypertension. Following his literature search (see Chapter 2), a deliberate decision was taken by the author not to use a medical screening model, that is, measuring vital signs and using other diagnostic tests such as urine and blood analysis. The finding of three cases of hypertension may suggest that the measuring of some basic vital signs such as blood pressure might be appropriate in future work.

One resident was found to have schizophrenia. This had not been a part of the project nurse's referral as he confined himself to descriptions of the resident's presenting mental state as opposed to attempting a psychiatric diagnosis. In this case, however, the GP knew the patient's previous history.

The GPs were asked whether they had looked after hostel residents before. All of them had, one running regular clinics for the homeless in a local hostel and regularly visiting men in other hostels. They were then asked their views about the delivery of an effective service for hostel residents.

It was obvious from their replies that most of the GPs had given the problem of delivering care to the homeless considerable thought. Of particular interest to the author was the number who expressed the need for effective access to general practice (10) – an 'open door' policy of registering any resident onto the practice (7) – as part of a service integrated into the mainstream primary health-care services (8). None of the GPs considered that these patients should be looked after by somebody else, for example a specialist medical team. This was interesting because much of the literature describes specialist medical projects (Powell 1987b, El Kabir et al 1989).

Five GPs, however, thought that specialist health staff should be available to meet the needs of some vulnerable individuals, in particular the mentally ill and the elderly. Most of the GPs thought that homeless people had the potential to acquire a good service in Glasgow, although some believed that the health provision for this group could be better co-ordinated. Six GPs made particular mention of the importance of having sympathetic hostel staff. One of them said that in one hostel (not in the study), staff were unhelpful and that this made it difficult for him to find and keep contact with his patients.

It was also made clear by 10 GPs how difficult it was to provide care for this group, the difficulty the GPs had following through a plan of action being highlighted. One doctor gave the example of how a man might attend his surgery with a genuine problem one day, that problem then being diagnosed, but unless the man followed through the prescribed treatment or onward referral, it was difficult not to judge the original time spent on the appointment as a waste of time for both the GP and the man himself.

The effect of the hostel environment on an individual's motivation was recognized by the majority of the GPs. They acknowledged how a poor environment might have a negative effect on motivation and that there may also be a brutalizing effect on the men.

Two GPs commented that some men appeared to 'take a drink' to give them the courage to visit the health centre and said how inarticulate this practice made them. Nine of the GPs also commented that residents sometimes attended the GP's surgeries in a drunken state.

Only one of the GPs was openly judgemental of this group. He talked about the men as 'this class of person' and how 'one doesn't expect to give them the same treatment'. Even when talking about the men's alcohol abuse, the other GPs were not critical, merely stating how disadvantageous this was to the individual. Apart from this singular exception, none of the GPs complained about the men disrupting the health centre or other patients.

Discussion

The author's general impression, therefore, on completion of the interviews, was of a group of GPs who genuinely believed that the care of hostel residents should be provided by the primary health-care team, with specialist intervention for recognized vulnerable individuals. The facility to achieve this belief was already in place, but the process needed more focused co-ordination. Part of a co-ordinated service, some GPs suggested, could include the ongoing monitoring of the residents. An opportunity to do so was already present as many of the residents attend regularly for sickness certificates.

There could, however, be practical difficulties, such as non-attendance, combined with a poor clinical outcome if residents did not take up onward referrals and prescribed treatments. This last point seemed to have the most profound effect on the actions of the GPs. This was seen particularly in relation to referrals for depression – none of the men referred as a result of a high HAD Scale depression score were treated, giving a general impression that the GPs responded to the men, possibly from a sense of moral obligation, while feeling that the situation was, in most cases, clinically hopeless because the men's lifestyle and environment militated against a satisfactory outcome. The assumptions behind this attitude will be discussed in Chapter 9.

The CPN

Thirty-one men were referred by the project nurse to the CPN. The CPN service to hostels for the homeless had only recently begun when this study was operating. Table 6.3 summarises the results of these referrals. The project nurse made no attempt to make a specialist diagnosis but referred the men if they presented with expressed psychological problems, if they displayed bizarre behaviour and/or if their HAD Scale score, particularly for depression, was high. A high level of anxiety was reported if it was combined with other signs and/or symptoms.

Eighteen men were seen by the CPN, who made 11 specialist referrals, none of which would have been made directly by the project nurse working solely on his own authority. These 11 referrals were made with a view to resolving the individual's psychiatric illness.

Conversely, the CPN described the 'ongoing monitoring' of 10 patients as part of the process that she was initiating to build up a caseload of vulnerable individuals who would require attention for the

Table 6.3: Community psychiatric nurse (CPN) responses to 'What did you do as a result of the nursing referral you received regarding this resident?'.

	Number of residents
Ongoing monitoring	10
Referred to consultant geriatrician	1
Appointment for alcohol detoxification	2
Accompanied patient to psychiatrist	2
Referred to psychiatric hospital	3
Alcohol project advice	2
Referred to mental handicap team	1
Not seen by the CPN – no action	12
Patient in prison – no action	1

period of their stay in hostel accommodation, not necessarily with a view to clinical resolution and discharge, but in a way more comparable to that of the health visitor model of monitoring vulnerable families.

All of the men referred by the project nurse and seen by the CPN received some form of ongoing input from the CPN team and other mental health services. Thirteen of the men were not seen by the CPN because they were no longer resident when she tried to find them. This reflects the fact that there was some delay between the referral by the project nurse and action by the CPN. The CPN was in the initial stages of her project, and she and the project nurse had to negotiate methods of communication.

The CPN made special mention of seven men who presented with particular factors that influenced her actions. These were a resident who had suffered a recent bereavement, a withdrawn resident, one suffering from delusions, a resident she considered suicidal, a known schizophrenic and a resident who was mentally handicapped. One resident she considered hypochondriacal, although she still considered him to be vulnerable and in need of ongoing monitoring.

Three of the seven men presented difficulties to the CPN. One patient was difficult to find because the project nurse had given the wrong name – the patient was difficult to understand, and the project nurse had heard him incorrectly. One man denied experiencing hallucinations despite displaying some bizarre behaviour. This made referral to the psychiatrist difficult, as a minimal degree of compliance and co-operation was necessary to make a correct diagnosis and prescribe subsequent treatment.

The CPN commented on the poor general health state of the men referred and the effect of this poor physical state on their mental well-being, as well as vice versa. The main difficulty, in her opinion, lay in identifying the psychiatric and other health problems and planning a course of action. Psychiatric assessment was made difficult when two men were found to be drunk or under the influence of drugs at the time of her visit.

The CPN reported that four of the referrals were inappropriate, as two had already been seen by the psychiatrist and two were not, in her opinion, mentally ill. However, she accepted that the project nurse, as a generic district nurse, was not in a position to make such decisions. This again highlighted the role of the district nurse as a generalist, sometimes making specific referrals to other agencies, but also making some referrals in order to obtain a specialist second opinion. This point will be discussed further in Chapter 10.

Hypertension was detected by the CPN in one man, and another man she diagnosed as mentally handicapped rather than mentally ill. The CPN reported that this man demonstrated how vulnerable individuals in an environment such as a hostel often presented with similar problems, and that professionals had to place diagnostic labels on the individual to ensure ongoing care.

The CPN had looked after homeless residents before and, when asked her views on the delivery of an effective service to them, stated that she considered the most important factor to be the clarification of roles between the different health and social care providers. Once this was achieved, more specific and appropriate referrals could be made. This was particularly important between different nursing services, she stated.

The author noted how the CPN's priorities for case-finding centred around the identification and protection of psychotic patients. Residents with depression or anxiety were considered to be more able to care for themselves, and she saw the role of the CPN in these cases as reactive, that is, responding to the residents' requests for assistance. The CPN stated that depression would be difficult to treat in the hostels because, in her opinion, the poor environment played a major part in the men's ability to achieve a positive outcome; in other words, she was doubtful that the men would respond well to medical treatment while living in the hostels.

When asked why diagnosed psychotic patients were treated differently, that is, why they were proactively sought, she stated that these patients were considered by psychiatrists to be more of a priority and were less able to make informed decisions and choices for themselves than were patients with depression. These priorities and assumptions will be discussed further in Chapter 9 and their service implications in Chapter 10.

The final point made by the CPN related to the need to reconsider the criteria for placing psychiatrically ill residents under a 'Section' within the terms of mental health legislation. She had noticed how difficult it was to get seriously ill residents into hospital. Part of the problem appeared to be that hospital agencies considered hostels to be on a par with other forms of accommodation and made no special allowances for men living in these circumstances. The project nurse found a similar attitude from hospitals providing care for physically ill men in relation to their discharge policy.

Discussion

The interview with the CPN demonstrated a difference in emphasis between the approach of the project nurse and the priorities of the CPN. The project nurse was seeking to access services that would improve the mental state of residents, particularly those who demonstrated signs of biogenic depression.

The CPN, however, expressed her priority to be seeking residents with psychotic illness who needed ongoing monitoring and protection and, in some cases, appropriate hospital care. She appeared to have a similar attitude to many of the GPs, considering that conditions such as depression were difficult to resolve because health professionals could make so little difference to the men's living environment, which she considered to be central to the mental state of those residents who were depressed.

It was also apparent that her approach was much more focused than that of the project nurse; that is, she was screening for specific manifestations of psychiatric morbidity, whereas the project nurse included social, welfare, nursing and medical needs in his assessment. This is not a criticism but an observation that highlights the different functions or roles undertaken by the district nurse and the CPN, both in terms of this study and possibly in the general field of practice. The service implications of these different approaches will be discussed in Chapter 10.

District nurses

Referrals

As the project nurse undertook the assessments of the residents, he – and the author – had no preconceived expectations or estimations of the probable number of men who would require referral to a district nurse. After the first few weeks of the study, the project nurse expressed his worry that so few men were being referred. It may be seen from the residents' identification numbers in the following exposition that the six residents referred were spread evenly throughout the fieldwork period.

It was during the fieldwork that it became obvious to both the author and the project nurse that two distinct roles were possible for district nurses in particular and community nurses in general. The project nurse was acting as a case-finding proactive generalist and making specific referrals to his district nursing colleagues. The district nurses acted as reactive specialists to the referrals; that is, they responded to a defined field of physical conditions in the same way as they responded to referrals from hospital and community medical sources.

It should be emphasized at this stage that whereas the author and project nurse were aware in a general way (from their own practice and from the literature) of these two roles, it was only during the course of the study that the dramatic difference between these two roles became apparent, as did the possible service implications for patterns of practice. This difference is arguably the most important finding of the study.

There was a striking difference between the great variety of interventions (treatments, referrals and advocacies) carried out by the project nurse in his role and the limited interventions carried out by the district nurses responding to the project nurse's referrals. In Chapter 7, a further examination will take place, these district nurses' actions being compared with the actions considered by an expert panel to be the most probable responses that district nurses would make.

Information from the project nurse's incident diary regarding the referrals of six residents to five district nurses will now be presented, followed by the responses made by the district nurses to the author in their interviews with him.

Resident 1

Case ID: 010; district nurse ID: 101

On examination by the project nurse, the resident was unable to state his name, date of birth, age or location. He was not registered with a GP. He scored 1 out of 10 on the Mental Status Questionnaire and appeared to be of low intelligence. He may also have been mentally ill. He was attended by the Social Work Hostel Team for help with personal hygiene. He was found to have bilateral oedema of the legs and varicose veins in his left leg.

Intervention by the project nurse: He was registered with a GP and referred to the CPN and the district nurse. The project nurse accompanied the resident to his initial GP appointment. In the referral letter, the district nurse was requested to assess the resident with a view to ongoing care and possibly long-term residential care.

The district nurse reported to the author that she had visited the resident three times and taught him how to apply the stockings he had been prescribed. The resident had been difficult to find as the wrong name had been given by the project nurse and the resident was a poor historian. The district nurse had found the resident to be confused, inarticulate, malnourished and frail. She did not think that the referral was appropriate as he was already being seen by the GP. She also considered that the resident should use the treatment room at the health centre for the care of his leg. No other actions were taken.

Resident 2

Case ID: 030; district nurse ID: 103

This 84-year-old man was found by the project nurse to have been resident in the hostel for 56 years. His speech was difficult to understand (he hailed from Romania), and his short-term memory was very poor. The project nurse thought that he might have been suffering from dementia. He appeared extremely 'institutionalized' and relied on hostel staff for food and cigars. He was attended by the Social Work Hostel Team and had recently been in hospital for bilateral oedema of the legs. He had refused to see a GP even after he had made a request to do so.

Intervention by the project nurse: This man was referred to the GP and district nurse for assessment for possible ongoing long-term care.

The district nurse did not visit. She regarded the resident as either a 'social or a psychiatric problem'. The referral was not considered to be appropriate as the district nurse never visited patients unless they were referred by a GP. In this case, she stated that the GP would not have 'let me go' because she thought that the resident had a history of violence.

Resident 3

Case ID:045; district nurse ID: 105

This 69-year-old man was assessed by the project nurse shortly after the resident had returned from Ireland. He had wanted to live there but had been rejected by his brother. This man was not registered with a GP. He was trying to stop drinking alcohol and had not had an alcoholic drink for 3 weeks. He walked with the aid of a stick and could not bathe unaided. An ulcer was found on the top of his left foot. His HAD Scale depression score was 14 (in the high range).

Intervention by the project nurse: This man was referred to the GP and CPN, as well as to the district nurse for an assessment with a view to the management of his ulcerated foot and for possible attendance for elderly care. The project nurse dressed the foot on two occasions as the district nurse did not visit straight away.

When the district nurse did not visit initially, the project nurse telephoned her. She informed him that the resident should be asked to attend the treatment room. The project nurse told her that the resident was unlikely to visit the treatment room, so she subsequently visited the resident and began a programme of treatment dressings for his foot. This programme was carried out by the enrolled nurse in the district nurse's practice. The resident was subsequently discharged when the foot healed, and no further action was taken. The district nurse considered the referral to be appropriate.

Resident 4

Case ID: 054; district nurse ID: 102

This 78-year-old man approached the project nurse requesting bandages for his hands. He was found to have contractures of several fingers on both hands. The project nurse felt that the man's his chest sounded congested, but the resident did not complain of breathing difficulties. Hostel staff reported to the project nurse that the resident needed a bath as he was incontinent of urine. The project nurse discovered from the resident that this was true.

Intervention by the project nurse: This resident was referred to the GP and Social Work Hostel Team. A referral was also made to the district nurse with a view to ongoing care and an assessment of his incontinence.

When she received the referral from the project nurse, the district nurse contacted the GP with whom she worked regarding the resident as the GP ran clinics for hostel residents. The GP had informed her not to visit the man as he already 'dealt with him', so no further action was taken. The district nurse did not think that the referral was appropriate in this case although 'usually it would be'.

Resident 5

Case ID: 071; district nurse ID: 102

At the initial assessment by the project nurse, this 60-year-old man appeared to be unwilling to impart any information, keeping his responses as short as possible. However, 8 weeks later, he approached the project nurse requesting a bandage for his right hand, which was found to have an abrasion on a skin graft site. The wound appeared to be infected and weeping. The resident was also found to have oedematous legs with partially healed ulcers. He informed the project nurse that he had visited his GP 2 weeks previously.

Intervention by the project nurse: The man was referred to the district nurse for assessment with a view to ongoing care, and for an assessment of his ulcerated hand and legs. The project nurse dressed the hand and his ulcerated legs.

The district nurse reported that she had made two visits to the resident and had dressed his hand and legs on two occasions. She found the resident to be 'generally well but unforthcoming'. She took no further action and discharged the man from her caseload when his hand had healed. The district nurse considered that the referral was appropriate.

Resident 6

Case ID:085; district nurse ID: 104

This 71-year-old resident received an assessment from the project nurse shortly after he arrived at the hostel. He walked with the aid of two sticks and complained of pain in his right leg following a previous fracture and arthritis. He had recently been an inpatient at the Royal Infirmary suffering from retention of urine. He also had a hydrocele and suffered from constipation. This resident's mobility was found to be poor, and he had difficulty getting into and out of the bath. He was worried because he did not have a medical card.

Intervention by the project nurse: The project nurse accompanied the resident on a visit to the GP, who arranged a day hospital appointment. The GP asked the project nurse whether he would accompany the resident to the Royal Infirmary as the resident had missed an appointment and he was suspected of having bronchial carcinoma. The project nurse thus accompanied the resident to hospital, where the resident was offered an inpatient bed. The resident refused this and returned to the hostel. He was also referred to the district nurse for assessment with a view to ongoing care and an appraisal of his mobility, urinary retention and dietary needs.

The district nurse visited the resident twice and arranged a visit for him to a geriatrician. She continued to visit him for 'ongoing monitoring' and had known him previously. She stated that she 'keeps an eye on him'. She had found the resident to be alert but physically frail, and was unsure whether the referral was appropriate as she 'already knew him'.

Summary and discussion

Three of the above six residents received specific district nursing interventions, one being taken onto the caseload for continuing monitoring. The two nurses who did not become involved stated that the GP did not think it appropriate for them to visit, one because the patient was thought to be 'violent', the other because the GP, who made regular visits to the hostels, was already seeing him.

The nurses who visited the residents made their nursing decisions mainly on the information provided by the project nurse. Two told the author that they informally 'kept their eye' on homeless residents. One of these nurses already knew the resident who was referred to her. There was, however, no strong evidence that the nurses undertook their own nursing assessment. In addition, none of the nurses enacted any networking or advocacy with other agencies or attempted to change the patients' environment and lifestyle.

The nurses tended to confine themselves to first-level minimum intervention, which efficiently addressed the main presenting problem but did not attempt anything further. From a discussion with the author in the interviews, the service appeared to be given in a friendly manner, although some concern was raised by nurses and GPs about women going into male hostels.

There was certainly some ambivalence among the district nurses about whether the referrals were appropriate. The most interesting feature of this was that appropriateness was questioned by two nurses because they already knew about the patient from another source. Having referrals from more than one source, and having knowledge of the patient from a previous interaction, was considered to be 'duplication'.

Another view of duplication, it could be argued, was that it was reassurance that one was well informed and 'on the case'. Such a view was not demonstrated in this study by the district nurses. Some of the GPs were, however, pleased to have the information as 'background' detail.

In response to the question of the provision of care to hostel residents, all the district nurses had cared for hostel residents previously. Two recognized that there was a potential role for district nurses in monitoring hostel residents, and another of the district nurses stressed that, to be effective, the work would have to be formalized and become part of 'official practice'. One district nurse stated that seriously and/or terminally ill residents were often referred 'too late for effective care'. Violence was not generally perceived to be a problem, but there was a recognition that some GPs did not like women going into male hostels.

The author and project nurse were both given the distinct impression that because this work was not recognized in record-keeping or in any other official form, it would remain peripheral to mainstream practice. There was a recognition by the district nurses interviewed that district nurses could adopt a generalist role, for example to help men who needed suitable accommodation, to assess and monitor groups, to run monitoring clinics and to provide holistic and/or complex nursing care.

None of them, however, actually engaged in these activities. There was a strong feeling that these matters were the responsibility of external authorities and that they, as individuals, were responsible for the delivery of focused, highly defined activities, such as wound care, which could address the difficulties the men faced in only a limited way.

Conclusion

This chapter has examined the responses of the GPs, the CPN and the district nurses to the referrals made by the project nurse. The health professionals interviewed took action and made further intervention in response to the referrals in some cases, and the information provided by the project nurse was thought by many to be useful. There was a general view that the clinical interventions of the study were meaningful, although there were some exceptions. The most striking features of the evaluation of responses are outlined below.

The GPs depended on people with special needs, that is, residents and their carers (including in this case the project nurse), to use the 'appointment in the health centre system'. 'Home' visits were for specific individuals with named acute morbidity. Only one GP visited hostels on a clinic/monitoring basis. The possibilities for monitoring were recognized, but there was a lack of incentive or formal directive and co-ordination to provide a comprehensive service to hostel residents.

What were seen as overwhelming environmental and lifestyle factors lessened the GPs' and district nurses' expectations of success, and importantly, there was as a result of this a serious questioning by them of the efficacy of interacting with this group. Neither group appeared to feel that group environmental and political advocacy was an important part of their remit as health professionals. Success, for them, was measured strictly within the confines of individual patient's treatment and compliance outcomes.

The CPN saw her main role as the identification, protection and care of the psychotic residents. Residents with other psychological problems were less likely to be sought out and would generally be seen only if they presented with a specific problem that they wanted to be resolved. Again, lifestyle and environmental factors were given as a barrier to successful resolution. There was a general assumption made by all the professions that much of the psychological morbidity, particularly depression, and physical morbidity was caused by living in the poor hostel environment. No one raised the question that some residents were perhaps homeless because of their morbidity. In Chapter 7, it will be seen that the expert witness (a psychiatrist) suggested that biogenic depression (indicated by a high score on the HAD depression scale) might be a causative factor in some men's progression to homelessness.

The responses from the GPs, the CPN and the district nurses indicated their view that the main cause of most of the men's problems was their accommodation and its concomitant unhealthy lifestyle. Little could be achieved because of this, so little tended to be expected. Thus, no special measures were taken to increase access. This assumption, to some degree, produced a self-fulfilling prophecy, the resulting non-uptake or non-compliance being attributed to the residents' choice.

All of the health professionals tended towards this environmental standpoint, particularly in relation to the men suffering from depression. The GPs and district nurses did not see it as their role to influence the environment or advocate for its improvement. As a specialist worker, the CPN was very active within the hostel trying to influence the environment. However she, like the other health professionals, did not try to discover whether residents were homeless because of their illness, which may have had an effect on the individuals' motivation and ability to respond to treatment.

It is important to emphasize that the author is not criticizing the health professionals or implying that they were entirely mistaken in their assumptions. What was interesting about the evaluation was the emergence of this strong professional group view, the implications of which will be discussed in Chapter 10.

Chapter 7
Evaluation: the expert panel and expert witness

In the previous chapter, it was seen how referrals were made to general practitioners (GPs), district nurses and a community psychiatric nurse (CPN). These health professionals were interviewed in order to discover the actions they had taken in response to the project nurse's referrals. Six referrals were made to five district nurses. These and the nurses' responses were given particular emphasis and discussed in detail. A variety of responses to the referrals were seen, ranging from specific treatment to a refusal to visit. It was also seen that the GPs and the CPN made no particular response to referrals made on the basis that the men had scored highly on the Hospital Anxiety and Depression (HAD) Scale.

This chapter will take the description of health professionals' actions a step further using two strategies. The first, the use of an expert panel of district nurses, was decided upon and detailed in the planning stages of the study. The second, the consultation with an expert witness, was agreed during the course of the fieldwork, following the initial responses of health professionals to the HAD scale highlighted in the previous paragraph.

The expert panel

During the planning stage of the study, it became apparent that the author and project nurse would be dealing with a number of individual district nurses, each of whom would be referred one (or a small number) of residents. These residents would be likely to present with a variety of problems, which would require a diversity of response. It would therefore be difficult to make an analysis based on the responses of a number of individual district nurses, each one of whom may have cared for only a single resident. An expert panel would consider six cases both individually and as part of a forum discussing them all. This method would provide a comparison of possible patterns of practice with individual cases and also provide insights from the group considering all the cases.

The district nurses were based in a small geographical area where there were several hostels for homeless men, many of which, including the Main Study Hostel, had been there for several years. It was considered, during the planning, that the presence of the hostels and the residents in that geographical area for several years might have affected the way in which the district nurses in that area responded to the residents. By presenting the cases to a group of district nurses who worked in a similar urban setting, but not in the same area, it was considered that interesting contrasts and comparisons could be drawn.

Six anonymized cases were presented to an expert panel of six district nurses, chosen at random, from a neighbouring Health Board in Scotland. The expert panel members were asked to examine the six cases, make short written notes (for their own use) and then discuss their findings as a group with the project nurse. The district nurses on the expert panel attended outside their working hours in a neutral environment (a church meeting room). Their discussion was recorded and transcribed, and forms the basis of the presentation and analysis in this chapter.

To test the reliability of this method, one of the cases (case 3) was chosen to be different from the others. Whereas the other five cases were all referred to a district nurse by the project nurse during the course of the fieldwork, case 3 received an assessment but was not referred.

The format of the presentation in this chapter of the work of the expert panel is as follows:

- Each case is exemplified separately. All have been given pseudonyms.
- The response proposed by the expert panel is juxtaposed with the actual response of the district nurse who received the referral from the project nurse. This is followed by the general responses of all the panel, with some specific quotations from the transcription made by individual members.
- The main points of contrast between the expert panel's proposed responses and the district nurse's actual responses to referrals are then highlighted.

Case 1: Written presentation to the expert panel on Mr Brown

Mr Brown is a 62-year-old man who has been living at the hostel for 4 years.

On examination, I found that he had bilateral lower leg oedema and varicose veins of his left leg. He was quite obese, which was something that concerned him. His general mobility was unaffected by these physical problems. At the time of assessment, he was unable to tell me his age, date of birth, the name of his GP or at which health centre he was registered. He scored 1 out of 10 on the Mental Status Questionnaire, indicating very poor memory. His speech was difficult to understand, partly because of his strong Irish accent. It was also clear that his understanding of verbal communication was limited. This made the completion of the formal nursing assessment impossible. Mr Brown attended his GP and was prescribed compression stockings, which he was unable to apply unaided. The Social Work Hostel Care Team was already attending.

Project nurse referral

I would like to bring the following details to your attention:

1. This man has recently registered with Dr B.
2. He has bilateral lower leg oedema.
3. He was prescribed compression stockings, which he is unable to put on.
4. He is attended by the Social Work Hostel Care Team for personal hygiene assistance.
5. He was found to have significant memory deficit.
6. I would be grateful if you would assess this man for district nursing intervention.

Actual response (unknown to expert panel)

The district nurse reported to the author that she had visited the resident three times and taught him how to apply the stockings that he had been prescribed. The resident had been difficult to find, as the wrong name had been given by the project nurse, and the resident was a poor historian. The district nurse had found the resident confused, inarticulate, malnourished and frail. She did not think that the referral was appropriate as Mr Brown was already being seen by the GP. She also considered that the resident should use the treatment room at the health centre for his leg treatment. No other action was taken.

Summary of expert panel response

All the members of the expert panel would have visited this resident, particularly because of his communication problems. They also mentioned how difficult it is to teach patients about compression bandages and their effective use. Compliance with medication, specifically diuretics to reduce oedema, was mentioned, as was the need for a dietician to assist Mr Brown with his dietary needs. Referral to and co-operation with psychiatric services and the occupational therapist were also mooted. A verbatim extract from the discussion from two of the panel members' comments represent the consensus view.

I just said I would follow it up, because the man's got quite a few problems. It's the fact that he's mental (sic); his status was quite poor. I wasn't quite sure just how – well you'd already said you'd had difficulty getting the history and everything from him, and I don't know that I would be any better at it – but I said I would certainly try, with patience. The main problems appeared to be his poor memory, the oedema of his legs and his obesity. The obesity could have a lot to do with his oedema, etc. Weight reduction could maybe have helped to alleviate some of his problems...it's awfully difficult to see how you can get through to him about these compression stockings. I don't know how we would get round that. I think probably someone would have to physically put them on for him. If that was us, fair enough, but if it was someone else in the hostel who could take over that job, then that's what I suggested we could do for him....I got the CPN to assess his mental state and I thought about a dietician for weight reduction diet, but I didn't know what the set-up was in the hostels: was there a kitchen that catered for them, or was that feasible in a hostel situation for a weight-reduction diet to cater for somebody? Those were my thoughts on the subject. (District nurse 1)

Well...assessing his needs because of his memory. I had arranged for a joint visit from the hostel team, who'd been looking after him for quite a while. They could let me know about his deterioration, how he'd been beforehand and his stockings...but I thought it was less of a problem so I'd referred him to the occupational therapist to hope that she would have one of those, I don't know what you would call it...[stocking applicator]...that would be best for putting on a support stocking. But with his lack of understanding, he didn't understand, and I kind of hoped that maybe after a few times the habit would help him to put them on so that he wouldn't go in every day just for that...and I sent him to the CPN....I wanted to check that he had the proper size of stocking to start with: if it was too wee, he'd never get it on. And to show him how to put it on, and to get him to show me in return to check his memory retention, and I wanted to contact the hostel care team to see whether they would assist with this patient. I wanted to know whether he was on diuretic medication and whether he was complying, and I thought I would visit him three times weekly to start with and involve the CPN with a view to psychiatric day care. (District nurse 2)

This first case produced a strong consensus of opinion among all the panel members regarding possible intervention, there being no specific differences. All of the nurses, however, expressed concern regarding the implementation of their care plan in difficult circumstances, particularly when these activities (regarding the compression stocking) could have a detrimental effect if imperfectly implemented. Compared with the actual response, there are similarities in that both recognized the need for monitoring and teaching the patient how to apply the stocking. The nurse involved confined herself to this specific problem, whereas the expert panel stated that they would provide a more complex service of multidisciplinary referral and monitoring.

Case 2: Written presentation to the expert panel on Mr White

Mr White is a 69-year-old man who has been living in homeless accommodation for 2 years. At the time of assessment, he was not registered with a GP. On examination he was found to have an ulcer on the top of his left foot; he walked with a stick (as a result of an injury to his right leg). He reported difficulty getting in and out of a bath. The ulcer was cleaned and dressed but required further treatment. Assessment revealed a relatively high score for depression using the HAD Scale. Mr White confirmed that he did feel depressed most of the time.

Project nurse referral

I would like to bring the following details to your attention:

1. Mr White has recently registered with Dr D.
2. He has an ulcer on the top of his left foot, which I have dressed with Granuflex.
3. He walks with a stick as a result of an accident affecting his right leg.
4. He has difficulty getting in and out of a bath.

Actual response (unknown to expert panel)

The district nurse did not visit initially. The project nurse then telephoned her, and she informed him that he should ask the resident to attend the treatment room; the project nurse said that the resident was unlikely to do this. The distict nurse subsequently visited the resident and began a programme of treatment dressings for his foot. This programme was carried out by the enrolled nurse in the district nurse's practice. The resident was subsequently discharged when the foot healed, and no further action was taken. The district nurse considered the referral to be appropriate.

Summary of expert panel response

All the expert panel would have visited this resident, treated the ulcer and taken him onto their caseload. They would also have assessed his need for other services. One nurse's testimony provides a summary of the discussion:

> I followed up this referral and I went to see him myself. He's...depressed. I felt I had to talk to him to get him to kind of trust me so that he would tell me any problems that he had and so that I could form a relationship with him. I would check his ulcer while I was in and redress it, probably with Granuflex, to see how it was doing, and assess his ability to get in and out of the bath as well as whether the bath aids would allow him to do it himself or whether he would still need help. I would assess his other needs – whether he had adequate nutrition for his ulcer, his sleep pattern, thinking about his depression there, incontinence and all the other things – and I thought about attendance allowance because he sounded as if he needed a wee bit of money to me. I said I would go in twice weekly for dressings but again it would depend. I would contact the GP, possibly to get a referral to a psychiatrist if the patient agreed and maybe medication to help his depression after he'd seen the GP. The CPN agreeing can act in conjunction with the GP depending on what the GP decided to do....And the occupational therapist for bath aids and an assessment in case there was anything else he needed.

Two nurses in particular concentrated on the Mr White's mobility and social interaction, particularly in view of his depression:

> I followed him up to assess his ulcer and his dressing requirements as well as his hygiene, mobility, nutrition, clothing to see that his shoes and socks were properly fitting and whether he had pain relief, and I was also going to contact to see whether he had any medication for his depression...I'd wanted to know if he'd contacted a GP. I would dress his ulcer twice weekly as my provisional action depending on

what he required. And the other professionals from physio to check, in fact now to prove, the condition following his old injury; I'd check his walking aid to see whether the height was correct and whether he was using it correctly. (District nurse 1)

I took up the referral to establish how bad the ulcer was...Also to assess how mobile he was because of an earlier accident that made him lame on the right-hand side, and this being his left foot I was actually wondering whether his mobility was decreased from the injury. How he copes with actually getting out of a chair and out of bed if he's unable to get in and out of the bath, whether the chair was too low and also any of the factors to do with falling. Whether there was anybody in the hostel able to assist the gentleman with bathing; if not, then social bathing (i.e. not undertaken by a nurse). Because of his depression, he doesn't communicate with other residents in the establishment (or would he maybe like to go to a day centre or pensioners club?); find out what hobbies he had, any friends that he had, why things would be a problem and why he was depressed. Something that he would like, to play bowls or go to a social club or whatever. I would visit two or three times a week. (District nurse 2)

This holistic approach was also seen as the expert panel made reference to 'contacting you' (that is, the project nurse), the GP and the CPN. Another nurse highlighted how she would examine the resident's personal hygiene facilities to see whether it was possible to make things easier for him.

The main difference between the proposed care and the actual response was that the expert panel members stated that they would become involved in activities influencing the resident's experience of daily living (washing, getting out of a chair, going to pensioners club, social interaction, and so on), whereas the the district nurse who received the actual referral, who did visit the resident and monitored the progress of healing of his ulcer, did not make any attempt to influence other factors.

Case 3: Written presentation to the expert panel on Mr Blue

Mr Blue is a 37-year-old man who has been living in homeless accommodation for 2 years. This man was referred to me by the hostel staff who were worried about his unusual behaviour. He was difficult to assess as his answers were often contradictory. During the interview, his eyes were constantly moving about the room (avoiding eye contact), and his facial expression was blank and unchanging. Mr Blue stated that he had attended outpatient psychiatric therapy; when asked the reason for this, he said that it was something to do with eating. He also said that he felt anxious and depressed at times. He described experiencing foot cramps when his feet were wet, pins and needles, and occasional numbness of both legs. In addition, Mr Blue reported that he experienced rectal shooting pains. On examination of his legs, there was no evidence of a physical problem.

Project nurse referral

I would like to bring the following details to your attention:

1. Mr Blue was referred to me by hostel staff who were concerned by his 'odd' behaviour.
2. During the interview, he did not make eye contact, and his eyes were constantly moving about the room. His facial expression remained blank and unchanging.
3. He gave a number of contradictory answers to questions.
4. He stated that he had the flu for 1 year and was worried about having a duodenal ulcer, although he had no symptoms.
5. He also reported physical problems:
   - He experiences frequent foot cramps when his feet are cold or wet.
   - He experiences pins and needles and occasional numbness of both legs.
   - He also experiences rectal shooting pains.
6. I have advised him to attend his GP regarding these matters.

Actual response (unknown to expert panel)

This patient was not referred to the district nurse but advised to visit his GP.

Summary of expert panel response

Only one nurse would have visited this resident. The other five would have contacted the GP and the project nurse with a view to linking the resident with other more appropriate services. One nurse's statement provides a neat summary:

> Well, I didn't go to this patient either. I got in touch with the GP to get additional information about him. I then got in touch with the CPN to see what she knew of him and to see whether arrangements could be made for her to see him, and I discussed the referral by phone with her, and that was about it. The only other thing I did say was that he experiences foot cramps, and his feet were cold and wet, so again I

got the social worker to give him the financial help to make sure he was properly shod to see whether that would help his physical discomfort.

The one nurse who would have visited this man appeared to feel morally obliged to see him. This is demonstrated in her response:

> Well I did take up the referral; I think I took up all the referrals apart from one. Although the bulk, I feel, of his complaint was mostly psychiatric, he did still have some physical problems. His pain, this is the one that had the rectal pain as well...I went and saw the patient, I did try to take a history from him but I got the same response – not really much eye-to-eye contact, etc., so that's where I felt that because of his depression and everything, I probably wasn't the right person to be there. So I went and discussed it with the CPN and also the GP to find out whether an investigation had been made to find about his rectal problems and also what could be circulatory problems, but on the whole I felt that it was more his psychiatric state, so I felt psychiatric rather than general nursing.

It is worth noting that this district nurse was not sure that she was the right person to do so, but she definitely felt that a health professional should see this man. This nurse and the other members of the panel clearly demonstrated the role of district nurse as expert generalist and advocate. That is, when confronted by a person who may not have been an 'appropriate' referral, they still recognized that he did have needs that could be addressed by other health professionals. Having made this decision, they proposed to contact the appropriate health professional and advocate his case.

As a reliability check, this case proved relevant. Five nurses would not have attended, and the sixth was unsure so visited 'just in case'.

Case 4: Written presentation to the expert panel on Mr Green

Mr Green is a 78-year-old man who has been living at the hostel for 25 years. He approached me looking for bandages to keep his hands warm. On examination, he was found to have contractures of several fingers on both hands, which made it difficult for him to put on gloves. When asked whether the contractures caused him any other problems, he stated that they did not. This seemed unlikely! Mr Green also suffered from dyspnoea, which he accepted was a problem on exertion. However, he also appeared to be dyspnoeic at rest. He had not attended a GP for many years and answered incorrectly when asked the name of his GP; this was discovered when trying to make an appointment with the GP he named.

Project nurse referral

I would like to bring the following details to your attention:

1. Mr Green has contractures of several fingers on both hands.
2. It seems likely that this would cause him functional problems, although he denies this.
3. He is dyspnoeic but does not appear to be receiving treatment for this at present.
4. He does not like attending his GP, which may explain why his problems remain unresolved.

Actual response (unknown to expert panel)

When she received the referral from the project nurse, the district nurse contacted the GP with whom she worked regarding the resident as the GP ran clinics for hostel residents. The GP had informed her not to visit the man as he already 'dealt with him'. No further action was taken. The district nurse did not think that the referral was appropriate in this case but 'usually it would be'.

Summary of expert panel response

All the expert panel would have visited this resident. Again, there was a demonstration of multidisciplinary networking. One nurse's statement represents the consensus. All the nurses recognized the difficulties that the resident might be experiencing with his GP and stated how they would try to engage with the man in order to help him through this problem and his general lifestyle difficulties, while also trying to address the breathing difficulties at the same time.

> I would take up the referral. I felt that his main problem was his dyspnoea and that that was the thing that had to be dealt with – the contractures of his fingers also caused him problems, but I think they were the least of his worries – so I would try to get him to see a GP and find out why he didn't want to see one. I felt that the dyspnoea had to be investigated and treatment had to be given, so I tried to get round him and tried to get him to agree to see a GP, and if he wouldn't go to see one, to see whether I could persuade a GP to go and see him. I also referred him to the occupational therapy department to make an

assessment again just for aids that might make things a bit easier for him. I also said that I'd probably go back maybe twice a week initially just to see whether there was any improvement in his dyspnoea and to see that a GP had actually gone, and that medication or whatever had been prescribed, and whether it was effective.

Two points arose from this case. The first concerned the thought processes of a district nurse when faced with a patient with obvious problems but no clear 'lead' for a way forward, and how she tries to get at what the patient feels and thinks.

Another nurse's testimony exemplifies the combination of simple strategies and actions with obvious concern for the situation and trying to reach an equitable solution. It is interesting to observe how she uses formal nursing actions such as assessment and ordering equipment but is also not afraid to act using her personal feelings. She argues with herself, presenting two sides to reach a balanced decision:

Well, I went to see him as well. It sounds daft when you read it out...I suggested putting the kettle on for a cup of tea because I thought that if I could get him to admit he had problems – because he wouldn't admit he had problems – if I could show him he had problems, then we could talk about it and get something done about it, and I could explain that if he saw the GP, he could probably do something about his hands and the breathlessness that came...check his ankles for swelling, and if he was passing urine how often.

I thought he'd probably poor nutrition because he's probably unable to cook, but again if he's in a hostel, they probably cook for him...I'd get awfully concerned about this wee man, so I had thought about meals-on-wheels and a home help, but again that probably wouldn't be relevant if he was in a hostel situation. He's probably not been sleeping well because of his dyspnoea, and I ordered him a back rest and more pillows and things.

I tried to get him to agree to a wash at least once a week. Just as has been said before, I tried to build up a rapport with him. If he wouldn't agree to see a GP or to have a GP come in, I visited him daily to build up a rapport till he trusted us to get him to see the GP – not for ever more, but I felt if even for a few days to let him know that he could trust somebody who'd monitor his diet and everything. I referred him, if accepted, to a home help, meals-on-wheels, the hostel team for bathing and the GP, and as a last resort I asked the GP to do a house call whether he agreed to it or not because I felt sorry for him.

One of the panel members was also concerned about this man and engaged in various activities to try to improve the situation. She also demonstrated how she would use these activities to gain long-term access to this patient:

> I took up this referral too, and found that this man needed a lot of help. I assessed him on the 12 activities of living, I tried to enlist a GP, contacted you to find out whether he'd been registered by a GP. I was going to use his dyspnoea as a reason for visiting him daily to assess him, an ongoing assessment, and to build up a good relationship with him. The only person apart from the GP originally was the occupational therapist to make a general assessment of the kitchen and cooking facilities. That was my original assessment. I would build on it.

The comparison with the actual referral in this case was very interesting. All the expert panel recognized the key role of the GP and stated how they would advocate the man's case in order to involve the GP. The panel did not know that the GP visited the hostels regularly (nor did the project nurse at the time of referral). In fact, the district nurse did not visit this resident but liaised with the GP, who saw the patient. The panel and the district nurse who had received the referral therefore arrived at a similar outcome, because of the special circumstances of that particular GP's relationship with hostel residents. The main difference, however, was that the district nurse who received the referral did not engage with the man and thus did not have first-hand experience of his continuing nursing needs, which the panel nurses, by their actions, would have been in a position to discover.

Case 5: Written presentation to the expert panel on Mr Grey

Mr Grey is a 71-year-old man who has lived in homeless accommodation for over 11 years, except for a brief period as a resident in a nursing home prior to moving to this hostel 3 months ago. At the time of assessment, he was registered with a GP in a neighbouring town, although he had previously been registered with a local GP. On examination, he was found to have a number of physical problems. He had bilateral lower leg oedema and arthritis affecting his right knee and hand, as well as chronic constipation, and he had recently received treatment in hospital for retention of urine. His mobility was limited by the pain from his right knee. He used two sticks to aid his walking. The [Social Work] Hostel Care Team had been attending this man in the past to help with personal hygiene.

Project nurse referral

> I would like to bring the following details to your attention:
>
> 1. Mr Grey is a new patient of Dr I.
> 2. He has a number of physical problems including:
>   – bilateral lower leg oedema;
>   – arthritis of the right knee and hand;
>   – walking with two sticks;
>   – constipation;
>   – he has been in hospital because of retention of urine.

Actual response (unknown to the expert panel)

The district nurse visited the resident twice and arranged a visit for him to a geriatrician. She continued to visit him for 'ongoing monitoring' and had known him previously. She stated that she 'keeps an eye on him'. She had found the resident alert but physically frail. She was unsure whether the referral was appropriate as 'I already knew him'.

Summary of expert panel response

All the expert panel would have visited this resident, and there was a general consensus on what action would be taken:

> I took this one up – this is the one in which I queried whether he had a GP, so I checked whether he had a GP and asked the GP whether he'd seen this patient because of his pain, his constipation and his oedema. I also want to see him and assess his pain control, constipation and oedema, and I also asked the Hostel Care Team to revisit him because they had in the past. In addition, I assessed whether he needed help with hygiene and made a referral to the physiotherapist, if the gentleman would let me ask for a tripod if his right hand was too sore for him to use, and also to help him with his mobility. I asked him whether he'd be interested in day care and, depending on the GP, whether support bandages for his legs would be appropriate, and I would monitor his constipation. I would ask the dietitian to give both staff and Mr Grey advice on a high-fibre diet. I would visit weekly. The professionals that I would call out would be a GP, physiotherapist, day care member of staff, dietitian and occupational therapist if appropriate.

Again, holistic strategies such as dietary advice were mentioned. Also apparent again was evidence that the nurses would try to improve his environment, as was the equipment to assist that process, such as a walking aid and the investigation of his financial circumstances. Concern was shown by two of the nurses that this man should not be in the hostel at all. One of them demonstrated in her statement how she would go about influencing his progress to more suitable accommodation:

> He's much better off in a nursing home than he has been in this hostel. So it was really to assess him, what his mobility was like, what treatment he was having for his arthritis and his oedema, whether he'd ever been seen by a rheumatologist, what his dietary habits were, what his fluid intake and output were, whether he had any physiotherapy, how much exercise he was able to do, how much of his time he spent in fresh air, how much time he spent just sitting around, what he had as a painkiller and how many he took...needed an assessment done for him for either residential or day care. I didn't feel that the hostel was the place for this gentleman.

The comparison with the actual referral in this case showed that the two were much more equal. Many of the strategies proposed by the panel involved engaging with the resident and his lifestyle so that they could monitor his ongoing welfare. The district nurse who received the referral was already engaged in these activities by regularly keeping in contact with the man. The panel thought that it was an appropriate referral, whereas the district nurse who received the referral was not sure as she felt that professional efforts had been duplicated. From the patient's point of view, however, the outcome from the district nurse who received the referral and the expert panel would probably have been similar.

Case 6: Written presentation to the expert panel on Mr Black

Mr Black is an 84-year-old man who has been living at the hostel for over 50 years. He originates from Eastern Europe and his English is poor, making communication difficult. He was referred to me by the hostel staff, who were concerned about his lower leg oedema and his complaints of painful hips.

Examination revealed that he had bilateral oedema pitting to mid-calf. He would not let me examine his legs above this level. I was unable to complete the formal nursing assessment as he was not prepared to co-operate. As a result of these observations, a GP visit was requested. In general, he exhibits obsessional behaviour and can become verbally and physically aggressive; his short-term memory is very poor. It seemed self-evident that he suffered from some form of dementia. This was confirmed by his GP.

A few weeks later, Mr Black was admitted to hospital as a result of worsening oedema and the formation of leg ulcers. A short time after being discharged, he was readmitted, having suffered a myocardial infarction. On discharge, his GP was again called out as he was complaining of chest pain, nausea and vomiting. A CPN had previously assessed Mr Black but is not currently involved. The Social Work Hostel Care Team were already attending to his needs.

Project nurse referral

Two referral letters were sent by the project nurse:

I would like to refer this man to you following an assessment by myself and would like to bring the following details to your attention:

1. This man is a patient of Dr F.
2. He was subsequently visited by a GP. He had been complaining of painful hips and had bilateral pitting oedema. However, he refused to let the GP examine him.
3. He also suffers from a form of senile dementia.
4. This problem is exacerbated by language problems as he originates from Romania.

Further to our telephone conversation regarding Mr Black, I would like to refer this man to you following a further assessment that I have made. I would like to bring the following details to your attention:

1. Mr Black has recently been admitted twice to hospital.
2. On the first occasion, his bilateral lower leg oedema had become worse, and leaking ulcers had formed.
3. On the second occasion, he was admitted having had a myocardial infarction.
4. He was discharged after 5 days and has been attended by Dr F since because of chest pain, nausea and vomiting.

Actual response (unknown to expert panel)

The district nurse did not visit; she regarded the resident as either a 'social or psychiatric problem'. The referral was not considered appropriate as she never visited patients unless they were referred by a GP. In this case, she stated that the GP would not have 'let me go' because she thought that the resident had a history of violence.

Summary of expert panel response

Four out of the six panelists would have visited this man. One nurse would have had a telephone conversation with the project nurse first; another said:

> I didn't go to see him at all. I went and spoke to the GP for all the information he had. We discussed him and thought he had so many problems he shouldn't have been discharged from hospital and hopefully would just go right back.

Three of the nurses would have visited on their own, and one when accompanying the general health professional. The consensus was that this man should not have been discharged and that he should be returned to hospital as soon as possible. The nurses would have used their networking skills to achieve this end:

> I discussed the case with the GP and CPN...then went to visit the patient with the GP – checked the patient out medically, and him having persistent chest pain, nausea and vomiting...readmitted him to hospital as he should have never been discharged into a hostel.

> I contacted the GP and asked him to visit...Meanwhile I contacted the Romanian Embassy Consulate or Glasgow University to accompany the GP and translate for him.

The singular point about this case is that when the reasons for action of the district nurse who received the referral and the expert panel are compared, they all agree that he should not be in the hostel and that they should not be trying to look after him there. The project nurse picked up on this point and attempted to find out some further details on how nurses decided on appropriate action. One panelist stated:

> I thought, well if it was really critical, you would have made a straight referral to the GP and not involved me at all...He shouldn't be in the hostel, and I shouldn't be supporting him there.

This point was at the centre of the difficulties experienced by the panel and the district nurse who received the referral. When the author interviewed the actual nurse involved, she was quite aggressive towards him, and certainly in the panel discussion, the project nurse perceived a similar air of vexation and uncertainty, as well as a general feeling of frustration. There was the recognition of a wrong without a clear path to resolution.

In response to this case, the panelists highlighted an important point, that is, the moral imperative to be seen to be doing something when one is provided with information. One cannot pretend ignorance, but what is the right thing to do? One panelist explained it thus:

> Once the referral's been made to you and you know about it, you're really obliged to respond in some way. I think that's probably why I went to see them all – because the referral had been made and you feel obliged to – although sometimes I think that if you were in the real situation, you might not always respond.

Conclusion

It can be seen that the responses of the expert panel provide an interesting insight into the probable actions of these district nurses. There was a general consensus, with some specific differences in strategy and action. Compared with the actual referrals, the main difference lay in the level of involvement on an ongoing basis. The district nurses who received referrals tended to confine themselves to the presenting problem. The second, connected, difference was the expert panel's proposed involvement of different health and welfare disciplines. These two differences combined to demonstrate what might have been a difference in philosophy between the panel and the district nurses who received referrals.

The district nurses who received referrals tended to take the residents' lifestyle, environment and health situation 'as read' and interacted with them only within those parameters. The expert panel proposed actions that would impinge on the environmental parameters, whether by involving a dietitian, advocating admission to alternative, more appropriate accommodation or referring the man to the physiotherapist or occupational therapist. This difference of vision aptly exemplifies the reactive specialist approach (of district nurses who received referrals) and more proactive approach addressing general health issues (that of the expert panel). A further discussion on this will take place at the end of this chapter.

It is interesting to observe that the expert panel were able to detect the case that was not referred, suggesting that their responses were realistic. Nevertheless, the actions of the district nurses who received referrals may simply reflect practical reality and the response to pressures of work, limiting their scope of practice. These points will be referred to again in Chapter 10.

The expert witness

During the fieldwork, it became apparent to the author and project nurse that the results of the HAD Scale questionnaire were providing both major findings and strong, negative reactions from the health professionals, particularly in relation to residents with high depression scores. When individuals were referred to health professionals and the results of the HAD Scale were presented, no action was taken. Three main reactions were encountered. These can be summarized in three quotations taken from the responses of some of the health professionals to the project nurse:

> Of course he's depressed; he lives in that terrible place.

> The HAD Scale was made for hospitals and is not relevant here.

> We are looking for treatable psychotic illness. These other illnesses are not treatable in these conditions.

The author and project nurse did not feel that they possessed the expertise to agree with or repudiate these reactions, although they did know from the literature that the HAD Scale had been used in a variety of settings. As the responses were a common reaction of health professionals who received referrals, it was important to present the HAD scores to an expert witness who could add other dimensions to the discussion.

It was decided, therefore, to present the findings to Dr R.P. Snaith, Consultant Psychiatrist at St James's University Hospital, Leeds, and originator of the HAD Scale. Following this decision, the author and project nurse visited Dr Snaith and interviewed him, presenting him with the reactions of the health professionals. The results of this interview are presented in this chapter.

The author sent Dr Snaith anonymized results from the statistical analysis of the scores from the HAD Scale questionnaire gained during the interviews with residents from the Main Study Hostel and Comparison Hostel. These comprised frequencies – how many men had scored in each of the three categories (normal, medium and high) – with the concomitant percentage relationships.

The author and project nurse visited Dr Snaith in Leeds and asked him, in a semi-structured interview, to comment on the findings and answer some of the questions that health professionals had presented to the author and project nurse. What follows is a summary of that meeting.

Dr Snaith began his response in the interview session by describing the development of the HAD Scale. It had been developed as a response to the high number of apparently depressed people passing through a hospital outpatient department and to the need to find some way by which to filter out those who were in need of intervention or treatment (that is, those with biogenic or clinical depression) (Snaith 1991).

The scale identifies the loss of the ability to experience pleasure, anhedonia, as the indicator of depression (Snaith 1992). When asked by the author about the relatively large number of residents found to have a high HAD score, Dr Snaith said that he was not surprised and described a situation in which someone suffering from biogenic depression becomes a 'flounderer', unable to cope with life, going from one crisis to the next and drifting into homelessness. He commented that these may well be people who have slipped through the health-care net, never having been diagnosed as suffering from depressive illness.

Dr Snaith went on to talk about the relationship between alcohol and anxiety, stating that although there was a relationship, it was not always obvious which came first. In relation to context or environmental influences on the HAD score, he stated that environment should have a minimal effect on the depression element of the HAD but a greater effect on the anxiety component.

Dr Snaith was very interested in the HAD (depression) results from the study. He thought that the relatively high number (approximately 14%) of residents who scored 10 or more was significant, the expected frequency in the general population being around 5%. He did not think that this could be explained by environmental factors and asked whether any of these men had been prescribed antidepressant therapy as a result of the study. When given the example of someone with a HAD (depression) score of 14, Dr Snaith stated that he would expect some form of intervention to take place for someone scoring at this level.

The term 'hospital', Dr Snaith stated, was used because the tool had originally been developed for use in hospital, but because, in his view, it was non-contextual, the tool could be used in most areas of practice. Dr Snaith was aware that the tool had been used in several studies in community or non-institutional settings and with different groups, for example:

- a study of Swedish mothers of retarded children;
- an Asian clinic study;

- a study into elderly dementing patients attending a geriatrician;
- a psychiatric outpatient clinic.

He considered that the HAD Scale was an appropriate tool to use with the particular sample in the study, that is, homeless men. He also stated that it had been used in a wide variety of environments and with widely differing groups.

Asked whether there were other validated tools that could have been used to achieve similar results, Dr Snaith cited the Present State Examination (Win et al 1974) as a possible tool to screen for psychotic illness. When asked how long it would take to administer this tool, he stated this would be approximately an hour and a half.

To return to the three reactions presented to the author and project nurse by the health professionals receiving referrals (shown above), the interview with Dr Snaith certainly presented another view. First, at least some of those with a high depression score would not, if Dr Snaith were correct, have been depressed because of their environment; indeed, they may have become homeless as a result of their depression.

Second, as Dr Snaith had predicted during his interview, there was a statistically significant relationship between alcohol use and anxiety score in that high impact of alcohol on lifestyle scores correlated with high anxiety scores.

Third, it would appear that the word 'hospital' is more an indication of where the tool originated rather than an exclusion factor, taking into account the evidence that the HAD Scale has been used in a variety of institutional and community settings – with success.

Finally, Dr Snaith stated that biogenic depression is a treatable condition that tends not to be influenced by environmental factors. The health professionals who received referrals based on the men's HAD score were pessimistic about the success of treating residents with depression.

The expert panel and the expert witness: combined evidence

After combining the evidence with the evidence of the expert panel, certain key features emerge.

First, there appeared to be an almost universal pessimism concerning the outcome of any intervention with this group. Expectations were low, and therefore even when clinical and other success might be possible, the opportunity to instigate treatment or interaction was not seized.

Second, the health professionals who received referrals did not, in the main, try to influence the structural or lifestyle environment of the residents, instead confining themselves to the immediate problem. However, the expert panel and the expert witness demonstrated strategies, such as treatment, referral, advocacy and admission screening for residents, that may have been successful in treating them and improving their medical and nursing care.

It would be wrong to end this chapter in an accusatory way. This study is not inferring that the health professionals who received referrals were not fulfilling their responsibilities. It has shown that other health professionals might have instigated other strategies, given the same circumstances. It has also demonstrated the potential level of intervention of which district nurses are capable with this and other vulnerable groups.

Chapter 8
Analysis: the men as individuals

In Chapters 4, 5 and 6, the results of the study were presented. In Chapter 7, some of the findings, specifically the responses of the district nurses, and the response of the health professionals to possible mental illness, were examined and tested against the responses of an expert panel of district nurses and an expert witness, a consultant psychiatrist.

In this chapter and Chapter 9, the findings pertaining to the residents will be examined further. This chapter will examine the men as individuals responding to their circumstances, and Chapter 9 will consider the men as part of a group, or subgroup of society. Both chapters will use a critical analysis approach, taken from the literature, to examine the men's responses both individually and collectively. Two main theories will feature: Roy's (1980) theory in this chapter, and in Chapter 9 a sociological analysis, including deviancy theory. These theories will not be used to 'prove' phenomena, as the subgroups demonstrating these phenomena were of limited size. Their function is instead to act as a pair of lenses through which the findings may be examined from different perspectives in order to assist the discovery of new insights into the men's experience and possible future action by health professionals.

Why adaptation theory?

In planning this study, the author became aware, from his previous district nursing experience and his examination of the five research projects reviewed in Chapter 2, that providing better access for homeless people to the health services was not the only requirement: other factors also needed to be addressed. First, there is the response of the health professionals to this group, and their assumptions. This has been discussed in the previous chapter. Second, there is the position of health in each resident's lifestyle combined with his ability to respond to the 'stimuli' that ill-health exerted on him and to the help offered to him, that is, his adaptive processes (Roy 1980). During the fieldwork, it certainly became obvious to the project nurse that discovering morbidity and making appropriate referrals (a broadly medical model) did not address all the difficulties encountered by the men.

To illustrate these adaptive processes and the difficulties that the project nurse encountered, three paradigms are presented below. They demonstrate that several of the residents, once assisted by the project nurse, did make changes to their lives. This contrasts with some of the negative assumptions encountered in the health professionals by the author and project nurse, in which a sense of hopelessness often pervaded.

A.C. was a 49-year-old man who had been living in homeless accommodation for many years. I first met him while assisting P.Q. to his room on the third floor. A.C. immediately became verbally aggressive and abusive. He stated that he hated 'f... welfare bastards!' P.Q. tried to calm the situation by saying that I was just helping him to his room. However, this did not help matters as Mr C. went on to say that 'These c... only want to help themselves.' He went on to tell P.Q. that it was his mates who helped him rather than the welfare.

I considered that, in this situation, my best course of action was to make a quiet but rapid exit. However, A.C. followed me down the stairs, continuing to direct abuse at me. On two other occasions, he interrupted conversations with residents by making comments such as 'Why are you talking to this w...? He's only out to help himself.' I concluded from our encounters that there would be no point in approaching A.C. regarding the assessment.

Over the next few weeks, I avoided contact with him as far as possible. It became noticeable that his attitude to me was changing when on one occasion he directed me to where I could find another resident I was looking for. For me, one of the highlights of my time working in the hostel came when he approached me, about 2 months after our original encounter, requesting some antiseptic cream for a laceration on his hand.

The importance of this paradigm is the way in which it demonstrates that some hostel-dwellers are distrustful of outsiders who come into the hostel offering a new service. Their trust has to be gained over a period of time by simply being there and being seen to help others.

Despite his initial verbal violence towards the project nurse, it may be seen that A.C. went through a period of adaptation towards the project nurse, finally placing some trust in him. Leading on from this comes another feature of adaptation, namely that levels of adaptation and ability need to be flexible to changing circumstances. Two further paradigms illustrate these areas.

P.G. had a number of problems, both physical and psychological: he was grossly overweight; he had bilateral lower leg oedema and varicose veins on his left leg; his memory was very poor (scoring 1 out of 10 on the mental status assessment); and his ability to understand was so poor that the HAD Scale assessment score is likely to be unrepresentative of his mental state.

As he was unable to tell me the name of his GP and there was no record of this on the hostel's computer, I arranged for him to register with a local GP. P.G. seemed unsure about attending for registration, so I accompanied him to the health centre. As a result of a second appointment, which he attended alone, he was prescribed a pair of compression stockings, although he had difficulty putting them on. This was a sign of the resident making adaptations following his interaction with the project nurse and the GP. P.G. rarely leaves the hostel, and from his response to the first appointment I had not expected him to attend future appointments unsupervised.

An assessment of B. revealed two problems other than his infestation with scabies. He complained of pain in his left leg; this appeared to come from the site of a fracture that had required internal fixation. He also had bilateral cataracts. He had attended an optician in 1991 and had been informed of this problem. Further questioning revealed that he had not consulted his GP on either matter and had not in fact attended a GP for over 6 years. I persuaded B. that both of these matters were important enough to warrant visiting his GP and arranged the appointment for him.

As a result of attending this appointment, B. received a prescription for analgesia and was referred to [Glasgow Royal Infirmary] for ophthalmic assessment. He subsequently arranged and attended a second GP appointment and attended the ophthalmic clinic appointment. As a result of this resident adaptation, B. is being admitted for ophthalmic surgery.

The project nurse observed in his notes:

Both of these paradigms highlight the difficulty some hostel-dwellers have in accessing the available services. This problem does not arise as a result of any barriers put up by the service but from the individual's inability to recognize that he has a problem, that there is treatment available, and that to gain access to this treatment generally requires attending a GP.

Having established that adaptations were made by some residents in the study, it becomes important to gain an insight into some of the factors that affect an individual's ability to adapt and respond. Roy's (1980) theory is used by many nurses as a model for practice.

The main precepts of the theory – the adaptive 'modes' (or areas of the individual's adaptive physical and psychosocial behaviour with which he can respond to stimuli) – are presented here in conjunction with data from the study. A critique follows that includes evidence of the limitations of adaptation, both from the study and from the social anthropological literature (Rapport 1993). In conclusion, implications for practice will be discussed, these being referred to again in Chapter 10.

As discussed in Chapter 2, Roy's (1980) theory views the individual as an adaptive psychosocial being, focusing on the individual rather than groups, although his interaction with society is deemed important. The rationale for this approach has been stated thus:

> Typically, nurses are viewed as caring for individuals. The recipients of nursing care may be an individual, a family or group, or society as a whole. Since the basis for any family, group or community is the individual, the discussion in this text will focus on the person. (Roy and Andrews 1991, p 6)

The individual is considered in four adaptive modes: physiological, self-concept, role function and interdependency.

In Chapter 5, it was shown how the project nurse used a reflective tool, modelled on Roy's (1980) theory, to assist him in assessing the needs of residents whom he had interviewed prior to intervention. This exercise was a practical application of the theory. In this chapter, as previously noted, the theory will be used as an analytical tool with which to examine the residents' responses and adaptations to their environment and health.

Unless stated otherwise, the tables used in this chapter are constructed from data from both the Main Study Hostel and the Comparison Hostel. Only statistically significant positive relationships ($p = <0.001$) have been selected. Attention will also be drawn to small groups of residents, represented in the tables, who displayed differences between what they said they wished to do and what they in fact did. These differences are presented as potential areas of tension and stress that may have a bearing on the individual's ability to respond positively to his health needs and level of adaptation (Roy 1980, Roy and Andrews 1991).

Adaptive modes

The adaptive modes are groupings of activities and behaviour that assist the individual towards the goals of survival: growth, reproduction and the control or mastery of one's actions (Johnson 1991).

Physiological mode

Roy (1980) recognizes that there is a basic human drive to maintain physical wholeness or bodily integrity. This drive motivates individuals to adapt and change their present behaviour, to seek assistance and to undertake measures to improve and strengthen their bodily integrity. Based on Maslow's (1943) Hierarchy of Motivation/Needs, Roy and Andrews (1991, p 15) cite oxygen, nutrition, elimination, activity and rest and protection as the 'primary needs' that motivate adaptation. These needs are influenced by the complex functions of the senses, the balance of fluid and electrolytes, neurological activity and the endocrine system – 'mediating regulating activity and encompassing many physiological functions of the person' (Roy and Andrews 1991, p 15).

At a very basic level, the hostel environment provides the facilities to enable residents to meet the five primary needs. The morbidity discovered in the study impinged directly on the residents' senses, balance of fluid and electrolytes, neurological activity and endocrine system. Specifically relevant were mental illness, substance abuse and old age. Many of the older men were found to be in a frail, compromised state. They were only just managing to cope, with the result that when they became immobilized with acute illness, their health very quickly deteriorated.

The project nurse was able to play an important role in assessing, treating and referring residents who approached him for help with physical problems. As has been seen in Chapter 6, many of the men followed up their appointments, although several did not. Many of those who did not do so clearly demonstrated some physical or mental dysfunction.

Table 8.1 shows the results of the project nurse making an approach to the residents and the subsequent intervention level. These results are compared with those of residents who approached the project nurse for help, who had a higher subsequent intervention level. Only 17 out of 106 of those who were initially approached by the project nurse subsequently required intervention, compared with two-thirds of those who approached the project nurse once, and all of those who approached him twice or more.

Two points are suggested by these data. First, many of the residents appeared to have a perception of their immediate health-care needs as the majority of men who made an approach for help to the project nurse needed intervention and most of those who were approached by the project nurse did not. Second, the study demonstrated that by making health and nursing assessments available, 61 men recognized that they needed help and made positive adaptations to seek assistance.

Table 8.1: Residents seeking assistance: Approaches by project nurse to residents compared with residents' approaches to project nurse

	Interventions	Non-interventions	Total
Project nurse approaches	17	89	106
One approach by resident	24	12	36
Two or more approaches by resident	25	Nil	25
Total	66	101	167

Chi-squared test, $p = <0.001$.

Forty-nine of these were found to need intervention. Table 8.1 appears to lend some support to the concept of residents seeking bodily wholeness.

The project nurse also found that whereas the men would often present with a specific ailment, for example an ulcerated foot, they would also express worry in terms of their life and living conditions. It appeared to the project nurse that these men were 'reaching out', using a single ailment in order to gain access to him and resolve more their general distress.

From a practice point of view, two slightly contradictory points emerge. First, it seems that if a service is provided in a hostel, it appears to help some of the residents, those who have recognized that something is wrong, to enact the adaptive processes and seek help, which may tip the balance in their favour. However, case-finding for residents who did not express a health need appeared to be less productive. As this was a research study, the purpose was to interview as many men as possible, but if one were setting up a service, this profile suggests that intensive continuous case-finding (as opposed to making a regular, more 'low-key' hostel service available for those who wanted it) would not necessarily be appropriate. The service implications of this will be discussed further in Chapter 10.

This pattern of behaviour, in which residents who sought help often needed intervention, was also seen in relation to the residents' use of accident and emergency (A and E) services. In Table 8.2, the relationship between recent illness requiring hospitalization and visits to A and E is presented. This relationship was supported by the experience of the author and the project nurse. They observed many men in a fragile and/or chaotic physical and mental state who attended A and E regularly and were also admitted as inpatients more frequently (as opposed to simply attending the department for minor trauma).

Table 8.2: Number of visits made to A&E in the previous 2 years compared with the last time the resident was an inpatient

Last time an inpatient	Visits to A&E				
	Never	Once	Twice	More	Total
under 3 months	9	6	2	8	25
3 months-2 years	29	14	10	8	61
3 years and over	50	7	3	7	67
Total	88	27	15	23	153

Chi-squared test, $p = <0.001$.

Much of this hospital attendance appeared to be alcohol related, but it was not entirely so. It will be noticed that the largest group comprises the men who had not been in hospital for over 3 years and had not visited A and E. The evidence from Table 8.2 suggests thus that most of the residents do not regularly use hospital services and that the men who do are a distinct subgroup interacting with the hospital on a frequent basis.

It would be foolish to overemphasize the importance of the data in Table 8.2, to 'overplay the hand', but it does appear to demonstrate men recognizing their physiological needs, seeking help and gaining admission within the context of the tight admission procedures put in place by hospitals. The table does therefore demonstrate that many of the men are indeed ill when they seek help.

Table 8.2 may also show that many men reach a physiological equilibrium over time in which they either resolve their dysfunctional state and/or adapt to their circumstances. In terms of the Roy's (1980) theory, this may be termed finding an acceptable level of wholeness and integrity. It may also demonstrate conditioning, with a lessening of expectations and aspirations. This last point leads onto the self-concept mode (Roy 1980).

Self-concept mode

The self-concept mode is related to the individual's opinion of himself and his experience (or lack) of control and engagement over his actions, as well as with his physical and social environment. Self-concept reflects the psychological and spiritual aspects of the person – 'the need to know who one is so that one can be or exist with a sense of unity' (Roy and Andrews 1991, p 16).

The consideration of the residents' perception of control over their actions and environment proved important in the study. Two very different groups were found. The first were men who saw themselves as hostel residents who were 'at home' in their hostel. These men often expressed an interest in improving the conditions, getting better services and making their life more pleasant, but they basically expressed an acceptance of their hostel resident status.

The second group were completely different. These men often saw themselves as homeless, going through a temporary period of rejection or 'falling off the tracks', or as being in a permanent situation that they would not choose and which was 'wrong'. These men wanted out, and hoped to improve their health and circumstances in order to achieve this end. Other men in this group appeared to have given up hope and saw themselves as being trapped in a place where they had been forgotten. Some of the men accepted that they were in the 'wrong' place and sought to get along as best they might in the circumstances. This subgroup were exemplified by men who accepted that their home was 'here' but who wanted to live somewhere else, and by others who had lived in hostels for many years, outwardly managing very well, but said that their home was somewhere else.

The project nurse noted this contrast between those men who, sometimes desperately, wanted to get out of the hostel and those who had made the hostels their home. Expressions of rejection were made by many men, often to do with their alcohol- or drug-associated behaviour, but also because of their residency in the hostel. Many men had overt low self-esteem with concomitant low expectations and service demands. In comparison, some men appeared to be content, pleased with their status in the hostel and the benefits of a communal, if limited, life.

Roy and Andrews (1991, p 16) recognize the 'physical self', that is, the individual regarding himself and observing 'I look terrible', and also the 'personal self', who can make self-ideals such as 'I know I can win.' The project nurse and the author interviewed many men who recognized their physical self. A number, for example, described how dishevelled they were, how chaotic their lives had become and how they missed their families. These men and others had lost or did not have the ability to overcome their present problems and were generally found in the group who did not feel at home in the hostel. From a practice point of view, considering the differences between the recognition of physical circumstances and of personal aspirations provided an insight for the author's understanding of the complexities of the group, particularly of the stress that this tension created.

Table 8.3: Where the resident thinks 'home' is compared with residents' ages

Age	In the hostel	With family/others	Elsewhere	Total
Under 25	3	15	7	25
26–50 years	17	25	15	57
51–70 years	36	23	18	77
71 and over	14	3	2	19
Total	70	66	42	178

Chi-squared test, $p = <0.001$.

Table 8.3 demonstrates how the family residence is perceived as 'home' by over half the residents under 25 years old but by only 3 residents out of 19 in the over 71 years age group. This is in contrast to three-quarters of the over 71-year-old residents who considered the hostel their home and only 3 individuals in the under-25 year age group. Noteworthy in contrast, however, is that in the largest group, the men aged 51–70 years, many of whom had been residents for many years, just under half considered the hostel to be their home and a third still considered their home to be with their families. Five of the men who were over 71 years, despite their age and adaptation to their circumstances, never considered the hostel their home.

In the largest group, the 51–70-year-old men, half of the men did not consider the hostel to be their home. It is suggested that this large number may illustrate a possible facet of compromised self-esteem and worth. Certainly, the author and project nurse heard many men speak of rejection by their families and by other groups and individuals. In terms of Roy's (1980) theory, this group may represent individuals whose self-concept and interdependency adaptive modes are severely compromised.

Conversely, it may be argued that this connection of the location of home with present circumstances is an overassertion, merely reflecting the fact that, in linguistic terms, different people mean different things by 'home'. At one end of the spectrum are those who feel 'Wherever I hang my hat, that's my home', and at the other those who perceive home in a familial, fatherland and spiritual context, as in the German word *Heimat*. Somewhere in the middle of this continuum lie those who always call the place they were born 'home'. How much importance an individual places on living 'at home' may determine how distressed and at odds with himself a resident is, that is, the stressors and tensions described in Roy's (1980) theory.

Taking these considerations into account, it would appear that many of the men were, to a greater or lesser extent, exiles from their base, and this would seem to support the self-concept stressors of rejection and feeling an 'outsider'. It also leads to the examination of the individual within the role function context.

Role function mode

Role function mode is connected with how the individual behaves and adapts as a member of society with duties and responsibilities, whether as a father, as a family member or in another role – 'The need to know who one is in relation to others so that one can act' (Roy and Andrews 1991, p 16). Role function is based on the integrity of social context.

In this study, the role function mode was demonstrated within the hostel community; six residents, for example, were noted to be caring for other residents in various ways. Outside the hostel, some men had other groups of friends and relatives in which they played a definite, if sometimes limited, role as father or family member. One of these roles was semi-institutionalized – a number of men lived in the hostels so that their female partners (the mothers of their children) could have the tenancy of the family home and gain single-parent benefit for the children.

Others with drug or alcohol problems played a similar family role, but, in these cases, this had been limited because of previous disruptive behaviour. A small group of men told the author and project nurse how, because of their past substance abuse-related behaviour, they had decided to remove themselves from their families altogether, considering this to be fairer to their children. This pattern of behaviour may also be seen as being indicative of low self-esteem, but the author certainly met two men who were in the process of building other networks in their lives in order to 'start afresh'.

These complex family roles of frequent, occasional or lack of contact were difficult entirely to quantify or explain. To begin with, each person demonstrated a different priority in terms of whether companionship with others or contact with their family was more important. Second, because, in some cases, the claiming of benefit was involved, residents were not as forthcoming as they were about other areas in their lives.

Some of the complexities of the residents' often ambivalent role within their families, and their living preferences, may be seen in Table 8.4. As may be expected, over half of those who said that their home was with their family stated that they would like to live with their wife or partner. Similarly, over half of those who said that the hostel was

Table 8.4: Where residents considered to be 'home' compared with residents' companionship preferences

With whom resident would like to live	Where home is			Total
	In the hostel	With family/ others	Elsewhere	
Wife/partner	7	22	9	38
Friends /others	36	10	11	57
By himself	24	33	19	76
Total	67	65	39	171

Chi-squared test, $p = <0.001$.

their home stated that they wished to live with friends, other residents or others.

What may be an expression of the tensions on the residents, however, is that just under half of the men who thought that their home was with their family wanted to live by themselves. Similarly, a third of the men who thought of their hostel as being home also wanted to live by themselves. If one considers how noisy and cramped hostel living is, it is not difficult to imagine how different an individual would feel about living in a hostel if he really wanted to live alone, compared with someone who wished to stay in a hostel.

The finding that two groups of men wished to live alone is supported by the project nurse's experience of some men who appeared to be desperate to move out of the hostel. These men lived side by side with men who considered the hostel to be their home and preferred other residents and friends as living companions (36 men). Roy and Andrews (1991) describe coping, and coping mechanisms, as being integral to the process of making adaptations. The hostel provided those men who considered that they were 'at home' with a completely different range of stimuli for coping and adaptation compared with those men who appeared to be desperate to get out of what they perceived was not their home.

Some men were therefore coping with hostel conditions that were in some ways acceptable to them. Others were 'tholing' or enduring the same conditions, which were to them hostile and the opposite of what they wished. The largest group (76 men out of 171) wished to live alone. Some were exiles from their family home. Others, especially some of the 10 men who thought that home was with their family but who preferred friends and other residents as living companions, may have been 'voluntary expatriots'.

Table 8.5: Where resident thinks 'home' is compared with how long the resident has lived in homeless accommodation

| Length of stay | Where home is | | | Total |
	In the hostel	With family/other	Elsewhere	
Under 1 year	9	27	5	41
1–5 years	16	20	15	51
6 years and over	44	19	22	85
Total	69	66	42	177

Chi-squared test, $p = <0.001$.

In Table 8.5, it may be seen how, in general, the focus of where home is moves from the family towards the hostel over time. It is, however, also apparent that 41 out of the 85 men who had lived in their hostel for more than 6 years still did not consider it home, in that half still focused on the family and the other half elsewhere. This table demonstrates a general pattern of adaptation towards circumstances. Adapting over time also appears to be combined with an area of possible stress and conflict with regard to the individual's role function as a family member, particularly for those men who do not adapt to the hostel as their home base, no matter how long they are resident.

The discovery of whether residents considered where they lived to be their home, supported by the nursing assessment, gave the project nurse insight into the individual residents' aspirations. This was helpful as it guided the project nurse in terms of whether to assist the resident in making adaptations (and/or receiving medical and nursing care) to improve his life in the hostel, or whether to place more emphasis on acting as an advocate to help the resident move out to what the resident considered more acceptable accommodation and companionship. The consideration of the residents' experiences, particularly this area of role function, in terms of Roy's adaptation theory (1980) thus had practical application. This will be referred to again in Chapter 10.

Also in regard to role function and to strengthen the points made above, Table 8.6 again demonstrates the residents' shift over time away from a family focus. Particularly stark is that only 6 men, after 6 years away from their families, wished to live with their partners and/or families. It is interesting also to observe that those who had been away from their family for less than a year had not made the

Table 8.6: Residents' companionship preferences compared to the last time the resident lived with his family

| Last time with family | With whom resident would like to live | | | |
	Wife/ partner family	Friends/others	By himself	Total
Under 1 year	16	0	12	28
1–5 years	13	13	19	45
6 years and over	6	41	42	89
Never lived with family	1	0	2	3
Total	36	54	75	165

Chi-squared test, $p = <0.001$.

aspirational adaptation of wanting to live with friends or other residents. They wanted to live either with their families or by themselves. The hostel had not yet become integrated into their coping and adaptive strategy.

Instrumental and expressive behaviour

Roy and Andrews (1991, p 16–17) describe how individuals demonstrate 'instrumental behaviour' such as caring for a baby, and 'expressive behaviour' such as cuddling the baby, as part of role function and linking with interdependency. As was described in Chapter 5, men were observed taking a specific caring role with other, usually frail, elderly residents. Acts of kindness, friendship and support were also witnessed, although it was also observed by the project nurse and the author that the social environment was generally 'hard' and sometimes hostile. Stealing, money-lending and other exploitative activities were present, for example. Thus, the cultural milieu tended to militate against open affectionate and expressive behaviour. Expressive behaviours, which in other contexts might be seen as evidence of instrumental behaviours, such as in a caring role, were therefore rarely overt. It would, however, be a mistake to deduce from this absence that residents were not involved in sometimes complex social relationships within the hostel community.

Interdependency mode

Interdependency mode (Roy 1980) encompasses the individual as an integrated community member, as well as any dysfunction that he may experience, such as rejection by others. Interdependency, in many ways, brings together some of the previous discussion as it focuses on the individual who is trying to become part of his human environment. Johnson (1991, p 386) highlights Roy's definition of interdependence requiring the 'close relationships of people that involve the willingness and ability to love, respect and value others'. In the context of the hostels, it is difficult to picture such an idealistic presentation of inter-dependence. However, the author and project nurse did witness residents' strategies to create community, and all too often the problem of the absence of community, namely loneliness.

Linking with the role function mode, Roy and Andrews (1991, p 17) assert that interdependence is based on affectional adequacy – 'the feeling of security in nurturitive relationships'. Two relationships support this 'adequacy', namely significant others and support systems. These systems are evidenced by the observation of receptive behaviour – receiving love and support – and contributive behaviour – providing love and support.

The project nurse found that his presence stimulated a focus for association in two areas. First, he 'collected' a small band of 10 regular residents who demonstrated considerable receptive behaviour. He also found five other residents demonstrating contributive behaviour by making referrals to him. The following paradigms provide a good description of both residents seeking help and their need for association.

D.J. was a 59-year-old man who had been in homeless accommodation for many years. D.J. became one of my regular customers. This was not because he had a particular physical or mental problem, but he had a frequently expressed and consistent desire to find alternative mainstream accommodation. To assist D.J. to achieve this, I advised him to attend the Social Work Department, the Hamish Allen Centre (the headquarters of the GDC's homeless services) and the local Housing Department Office. I made several phone calls to the Social Work Department, which resulted in a home-maker being allocated to his case. I also phoned the Hamish Allen Centre in an attempt to arrange an interview for him. Six months after I first met D.J., he was no closer to getting the flat that he so desperately wanted.

One of the major difficulties with this case is that D.J.'s alcoholism and his obvious inability to keep himself clean makes it unlikely that he would be able to sustain himself in a flat without considerable support. However, I believe that he deserves to be given the opportunity to find out for himself whether he is capable of living on his own, even if this only means giving him the opportunity to fail.

The paradigm above shows the chaotic distress of this man. He was aware of his needs but was incapable of making any adaptation, except to seek out help. His alcoholism, lack of control and loneliness contrived to disrupt his ability to function as an interdependent person. The project nurse found men in this condition difficult to help, as well as distressing to himself as a nurse, as he could not really enter into any effective form of contractual interdependency role with this man or others like him, despite a strong desire on his part to do so.

> H.S. was a 38-year-old man of Asian origin. This in itself singled him out from the other residents, but it was his use of the service offered by me which makes him stand out from the others. There were several residents who could be described as 'regular customers', but in terms of frequency of approaches he was my best 'customer'. This use of a health-care service is not unusual for H.S. as he is well known to the local A and E department and the receptionists of the GP practice with which he is registered.
>
> One reason for his heavy use of the available services is the pain he experiences in his right leg, which was injured in an road traffic accident and resulted in the knee being fused into a fixed position. This has had a considerable effect on his general mobility as he uses crutches to aid walking. His use of crutches appears to be a negative adaptation to his circumstances, as he should be capable of walking without the crutches. As he missed three clinic appointments over a short period of time, it seems likely that his dependence on the crutches has developed because of his failure to complete a rehabilitation programme.

From this paradigm, it may be considered that some of this man's difficulties stemmed from an inability to function in the hostel context. A factor influencing this inability may have been that the normal (for him) strategies of interaction and seeking assistance, emanating from his ethnic and cultural background, may have proved ineffective.

The importance of this paradigm, however, is that it shows how the resident, who had experienced physically disabling injuries, found it very difficult to relate to others and seek help effectively. As with the previous paradigm, this man found that his only adaptive strategy was to try to encourage the project nurse and others to love and support him, to 'look after' him, rather than to establish a reciprocal, more contractual, relationship (in which he would seek help and respond to advice before returning to the project nurse). This inability to create an effective relationship and to respond to the help offered was frustrating for both patient and nurse.

Of all the tables presented in this chapter, Table 8.7 is the most stark. It can be seen that nearly two-thirds of the men who scored highly on the anxiety score had been residents for under a year, whereas the vast majority who had been resident for 6 years or more fell into the normal category. The author and project nurse recognized the men's anxiety while interviewing them; many of the men expressed their loneliness and sense of instability as they tried to 'find their feet'. The expert witness, Dr Snaith, also stated that the anxiety score was sensitive to environment and that changes in life patterns do create stress. It might have been that, later on, the men either 'settled' down and accepted hostel life or were motivated to move out of the hostel.

During, what was, for many, an anxious first year, it was found that three-quarters of the men had visited their doctors, many of them on a regular basis (Table 8.8). Nearly half of the men who had been resident in the hostels for over 6 years continued this pattern of behaviour

Table 8.7: Residents' length of stay in their hostel compared with their HAD Scale Anxiety score

HAD score	Stay in hostel			Total
	Under 1 year	1–5 years	6 years and over	
Normal range	32	29	30	91
Intermediate range	15	9	4	28
High range	28	13	4	45
Total	75	51	38	164

Chi-squared test, $p = <0.001$.

Table 8.8: The last time residents were seen by their GPs compared with the length of stay in their hostel

Length of stay in hostel	Last time resident seen by GP			Total
	Under 6 months	6 months – 2 years	3 years and over	
Under 1 year	60	15	4	79
1–5 years	34	9	6	49
6 years and over	21	8	15	44
Total	115	32	25	172

Chi-squared test, $p = <0.001$.

throughout their residency, while a third of residents had very little contact with their doctor. This behaviour may be seen as the men, particularly the new residents, responding to the tension created by their single homeless state. Some try to change their circumstances by seeking to receive help and support, and enter into a nurturing environment. As time progresses and they build up more satisfactory interdependent relationships and ways of living in the hostel, some men cease to seek aid from their doctor whereas others will constantly 'cry out' for help.

The comparison of these two variables is of course affected by many factors, not least by those such as substance abuse. However, the author and project nurse observed this pattern of behaviour in the context of residents sometimes almost frenetically seeking help from and association with as many contacts as possible. This coping mechanism resolved itself with some men when they found a group or other individuals with whom to associate. Other men diminished their activities but became more solitary and withdrawn.

It was difficult to judge, either in individuals or in the group, which strategies were most successful. Nevertheless, the author and project nurse noted the number of men who engaged them in conversation and were left with a general impression of great loneliness among some of the men despite their strategies to associate with others.

What also became apparent with regard to the source of interdependency was the importance to the men of individual health professionals. The project nurse gained the impression that the way in which he interacted with individuals, that is, in a non-threatening and low-key manner, played an important part. The men also displayed to him specific preferences for individual professionals who came into the hostel; a professional's personality came under considerable scrutiny from the men.

Summary and discussion

The use, as an analytical tool, of the four adaptive modes of Roy's theory in this chapter has, it is hoped, provided some insight into the experience of the individual men in coping with and adapting to what may appear on the surface to be similar circumstances.

The physiological mode emphasized the drive of the individual towards 'wholeness'. Many men were certainly seen to be seeking out help and had been found to need intervention in most cases. Tensions arose when their ability to influence activity and self-protection were compromised, whether through substance abuse or old age, which also affected the senses and neurological function.

The self-concept mode was highlighted in that some men saw themselves as being 'at home' in the hostel whereas others saw themselves as outsiders in a transient, aberrant situation. Time appeared to influence coping and adaptation, but some men never lost their 'exile' status.

The role function mode demonstrated the differing roles of residents in their families and also the role function of the residents within the hostel. Stressors were again found, that is, gaps between what a man aspired to and his actual circumstances. Some men broke away from their previous lives altogether while some focused on their position in the hostel community and yet others made compromises, with occasional contact with their families.

Finally, the interdependence mode was sought by men both with each other and with the project nurse and other professionals. A need to associate with other human beings was encountered, as was the practical need for assistance. Some men seemed trapped by loneliness and an inability to make practical adaptations, which caused them to become caught in a seemingly useless cycle of constantly seeking association and help without being able to achieve anything and move forward.

The examination of the residents through the interdependence mode provided an insight into the difficult lives that many of the men experienced and into factors that might possibly affect the high level of morbidity witnessed in the sample group. Roy and Andrews (1991, pp 388–9) emphasize the importance of the ability to engage in both receiving and giving behaviours, 'expressing love' and 'providing physical and psychological support' cites how married men tend to live longer than those who live alone outside a close relationship (Roy and Andrews 1991, p 391). To support this assertion, Roy cites Berkman's (1978) Social Contact Index, which 'takes account of whether the individual is married, has close contacts with friends and relatives, belongs to a religious group or has organisational links' (Roy and Andrews 1991, p 391).

Through the consideration of the four adaptive modes, a picture thus emerges of some individuals who, because of their physical condition, including the effects of substance abuse, the harsh physical and social environment, their limited access to achieve a meaningful role, and their feelings of alienation and lack of self-worth, are unable to achieve 'wholeness' and a feeling of 'unity' with themselves or their social environment, whereas other homeless men have been able to create an albeit simple role and social context for themselves and achieved some degree of resolution and social integrity.

Using Roy's (1980) theory, it may therefore be possible to 'diagnose' individuals in the first, more dysfunctional, group in terms of a deficit or inability to achieve the full potential of the adaptive modes. This deficit may be seen in terms of an analogy with a human being's inability to exist without oxygen, food and warmth – his quality of life is also 'under threat' if he cannot interact, adopt a meaningful role and give and receive love.

This consideration of the study through Roy's (1980) theory has been illuminating. It has taken the examination of the residents, their physical paths to solutions, their human context and their health and lifestyle problems beyond the usually broadly medical model of causal morbidity and prescribed intervention. One related factor observed by the author and project nurse was the difficulty that health professionals experienced if they diagnosed morbidity without connecting their findings to the problems perceived and expressed by the patient. This dissonance often led to 'negative' adaptations or 'non-compliance' on behalf of the residents.

The use of adaptive theory emphasizes the need to consider how the patient's present circumstances are creating stressors for him. For example, if the main problem for the individual is that he hates being in the hostel and wishes to leave, it may be difficult for him to focus his adaptations on a medical condition diagnosed by a health professional, which he has not recognized himself. Another man, relatively content in his environment, may be able to focus on the condition and make appropriate adaptations to arrive at a resolution.

Difficulties with the application of Roy's theory

Two philosophical difficulties regarding Roy's (1980) theory emerged in relation to this study. First, the author and the project nurse found themselves working in a 'hand-to-mouth' world in which simply getting through the day was difficult for many men. In this narrow existential state, it was difficult to perceive the 'four truths' or principles of 'veritivity' on which the theory is based, especially the universality of truth and common purposefulness (Roy 1988). On a more practical note, it was also difficult to recognize the drive for wholeness and place, and distinguish it from often desperate instinctual self-interest.

Roy and Andrews (1991) recognize aspects of this problem of levels of adaptation. In some of her earlier work (Roy 1977), she hypothesized that 'levels of wellness would be greater with higher levels of adaptation' (Roy and Andrews 1991, p 452). Roy and Andrews found no evidence for this assertion in acute hospital settings, but 'there was such a relationship in the least acute settings and for longer stay patients' (p 452). These references do not directly relate to individuals such as homeless men, and they refer to 'wellness' in terms of the adaptations made as opposed to the inability to make adaptations as a result of illness or a harsh physical and social environment. In summary, there does appear to be a connection between level of adaptation and the ability to achieve a higher level of personal health and social integrity, although Roy's (1980) theory is not explicit on this point.

Second, Roy appears to make the assumption that areas of tension and stressors on an individual will motivate that individual into developing coping strategies and adaptations. In this study, many of the men recognized these stressors but were unable to enact adaptations, some because they were using coping strategies such as the abuse of alcohol, others because they were not capable of incorporating the remedies and activities suggested to them by the health professionals: the remedies appeared to be outside their normal range of movements and adaptations.

Roy's (1980) theory appears to infer that no situation is hopeless or untenable for any given individual as the tensions and stressors will create the opportunity to adapt. Whereas this may be a laudable moral principle, it has an effect of unreality in some situations. The author and project nurse found that many men were not in a position to adapt; instead, they had to endure, to 'thole' as the Scots say, and to absorb without changing or adding to their palette of coping and adaptive mechanisms.

Buck (in Roy and Andrews 1991, pp 290–1) recognizes coping strategies as an individual's 'habitual responses used to maintain a state of adaptation'. She also recognizes that the 'disruption of any of these [responses] and other routines might threaten the person's sense of physical self'(p 291). In terms of some of the residents, these two observations may provide an insight into a fundamental problem. If the individual's usual coping strategy is not to adapt but to endure and absorb, then to encourage him to make adaptations, even ones with positive benefits, may cause damage to his self-integrity.

This endurance could be observed either when the resident did not have the adaptive mechanisms or when the situation that the resident faced was so personally disastrous as to be irresolvable, at least in the short to medium term. This could be seen with terminal illness, irretrievable relationship breakdown and chronic mental illness. The author and project nurse found that, in general, the residents had very few coping and adaptive skills, which may have been part of the reason that they were resident in the hostel in the first place.

The hostel environment

The possible lack of coping and adaptive skills among the men may have been influenced by a hostel environment that did little to augment the meagre strategies used by this vulnerable group. Roy's

(1980) theory does not appear to give any insight into the influence of structural environment. Definitions of environment are focused on the more 'micro' physiological environment, for example 'Many environmental stimuli influence the process of protection – eg perspiration [is influenced by] ... room temperature' (Roy and Andrews 1991, p 154). The environment is thus considered to be a positive force. Roy and Andrews (1991) continue:

> As the environment changes, the person has the continued opportunity to grow, to develop and to enhance the meaning of life for everyone...The changing environment stimulates the person to make adaptive responses.

Reiterating an earlier point, Roy's assertions, in terms of the residents' living environment, appear to be based on the assumption that the ability to adapt is boundless and translates to every environmental context. Whereas this may be witnessed in 'mainstream' settings, this study, and the literature regarding other marginalized groups described in Chapter 2, would dispute this assumption.

Other work – a social anthropological perspective on coping strategies

The author decided to investigate literature from another academic discipline in relation to the apparent lack of coping and adaptive mechanisms. In the social anthropological field, Rapport (1993) undertook a study in a village in the English Lake District. In it he interviewed various villagers, observing their views and the processes by which they interacted with their changing circumstances. When Rapport began the interviews, it appeared to him that the individuals responded and adapted to different events in a variety of ways, seemingly taking each event and making the (in their eyes) appropriate responses. As the study progressed, however, he discovered that these responses actually formed a 'loop'.

In a casual or short-term encounter, it seemed that the variety of responses constituted an adaptation to different circumstances, but in the longer term, individuals were found to have a loop of responses that were used all the time. Some people had longer loops than others, but a repetition of response was eventually always discovered. This view contrasts with Buck's assertion, cited above, that these 'habitual responses' were a prerequisite for the maintenance of a state of adaptation.

The relevance of Rapport's (1993) work to the present study was that this observation of limited mechanisms had resonance with the experience of the author and the project nurse, in which many of the men displayed extremely short 'loops' of response, coping and adaptive processes. Perhaps as part of the longer-term monitoring of patients, it should be accepted by nurses, in a more formal way, that adaptation may not be possible in all cases.

Conclusion

Despite possible areas of contention in the founding assumptions of Roy's (1980) theory, an analysis of some of the data using the four adaptive modes has had the practical effect of highlighting important facets of the individual residents' experiences. This is particularly so as each resident attempts to make sense of his physical, psychological and human environment and take appropriate actions to seek assistance and help himself. It was, however, also seen that residents, as a group, seemed to be affected by external factors over which they had little control. These will be examined more closely in Chapter 9.

Chapter 9

Analysis: the residents as a group

The previous chapter provided a framework for and insight into the residents' individual responses and adaptations to their environment, health and health services. This chapter will have a sociological focus, using themes from the literature that include deviancy theory and professional interaction with groups of marginalized people. The chapter will exemplify and discuss evidence that provides an insight into the residents as a group and the lifestyle choices they made.

A sociological perspective is relevant to this study as it places the residents within the context of society at large, as well as providing information on some of the dynamics of the residents as a group. Of relevance also is that the author, as a nurse, has a professional tendency to consider patients as individuals. Considering the group as a whole may provide the study with a more comprehensive analysis of the data.

Chapter 2 highlighted the view that deviancy theory was not a unified school of thought but a diverse range of perspectives that shed light on how dominant groups and subgroups interacted within a societal or institutional context, in particular how certain groups displayed signs of dependency and loss of individuality (depersonalization), as well as demonstrating antisocial, rule-breaking or deviant behaviour.

Groups and subgroups

Groups are described living outside the norms of the dominant society (Goffman 1961, Kaplan 1991). In the deviancy theory literature, there are descriptions of groups of men and the influences of their family, employment and upbringing as they progress through life. Sampson and Laub (1990) describe a 'trajectory' of development through childhood and into adulthood, especially 'work life, marriage, parenthood, self esteem and criminal behaviour' (p 610). The data amassed in this study demonstrate how many residents have become sometimes entirely separated from these influences and also engage in criminal behaviour.

The hostel resident group

It has been argued that an individual's progression through life is influenced by 'transitions', or formative life events. Thus, for example, events such as marriage and starting work may be considered to have a stabilizing effect on individuals that influences their behaviour in later life, whereas other events, such as imprisonment, may be said to be destabilizing. In particular, these transitions may affect future criminal or deviant behaviour. The focus of this study has been on a group of men who were generally older than those people usually studied by writers in the deviancy tradition, whose work has tended to assume that there is a natural decline in an individual's deviant behaviour as he gets older (Hirschi and Gottfredson 1983).

This study also differs from many deviancy studies as it presents simply a 'snapshot' of a population of men at a particular period in time. The study of the deviancy literature has, however, provided insights into the behaviour of some of the residents as a group, as it places their behaviour and responses into context with other groups, particularly marginalized people.

The purpose of this chapter is not to prove or disprove the assertions of deviancy theory. However, there does appear to be evidence to show that the residents should be studied as a group influenced both by social and developmental factors such as their relationships, living preferences and criminal behaviour, and also by individual sets of circumstances or events that affect their patterns of future behaviour.

Knight et al (1977) studied a group of Borstal boys from adolescence into adulthood and found that whereas marriage did not lessen criminal activity, it did reduce antisocial behaviour such as drunkenness and drug-induced activities. Given that single homeless residents are, by definition, not in these possibly stabilizing relationships, and that they are also associated with antisocial behaviour, this chapter will examine, with exemplars from the data, factors regarding their group behaviour. These may provide some explanation of the rationale, if any, of living in single homeless accommodation.

Relevance of place: the hostels as institutions

Another sociological study examined the 'existential significance of places' (Godkin in Buttimer and Seamon 1980, p 73) in terms of 'rootedness and uprootedness'. The study stated that the space one inhabits has a defining influence on the individual's and group's view of themselves. The study also suggests that a place can elicit shared 'meanings and common symbols' in groups and influence their response to and interactions with the world.

Considering the position of single homeless residents living in a hostel, this chapter will explore the evidence of the residents' belonging to and alienation from the hostels and society, and highlight differences between subgroups within the hostel community.

Two main subgroups

Attention is drawn to two main subgroups, who demonstrate opposing attitudes regarding their sense of belonging in relation to the hostels. One group were 'at home' in the hostels and appeared to demonstrate a distinct, shared, subcultural identity, preferring the companionship of other residents to that of family or outside individuals. The other group were not 'at home' in the hostels, demonstrated conflicting responses to their circumstances and would have preferred to live outside the hostels, either with their families or alone.

The purpose of this exploration is to provide an insight into the reasons for the hostels being there, demonstrating their functional role together with evidence of the residents' experience of hostels and the rationality of their actions, that is, what they wanted from hostels. The exploration is therefore of the external conditions and individual responses. It is also an examination of some of the group dynamics emanating from the residents' shared interpretations of and values held in relation the hostel setting.

Implications of the study of group dynamics for practice

Service delivery issues will be discussed, particularly in relation to some residents adopting a passive role with regard to their personal and health needs, as will nurses' moral judgement on these decisions. The ambivalence that this judgement creates for nurses providing reactive care – as first aid or rescue, for expressed need only or in a more proactive holistic approach – to identified, sometimes unexpressed need will be highlighted.

This chapter will thus consider elements of the residents' behaviour and experience that help to explain whether the men have made a choice to live as they do or whether the situation of hostel living is forced upon them. Redhead (in Abrams and Brown 1984, p 294) presents the 'traditional dichotomy' of deviancy:

> *either* deviants have the capacity of free will and make rational choices to behave in an irrational fashion, *or* they are determined or propelled into such action, through no fault of their own by internal or external factors.

In terms of this study, Chapter 8 has examined individual choices and adaptations. By examining individuals, subgroups and the hostel group as a whole, this chapter will present a sociological perspective including deviancy theory, specifically considering rule-breaking, itinerant disorganized lifestyles, group values and norms, conflict and co-operation, internal and external barriers, and functionalism (positive and negative rationales for the hostels' existence). Finally, the chapter will highlight the attitudes of health professionals and others towards this and other marginalized groups.

Rule-breaking: 'ex-prisoner' and 'non-prisoner' subgroups

Rule-breaking is a primary feature of deviancy theory. As highlighted in Chapter 2, subgroups are seen to live separately from the main society and behave in a deviant or aberrant manner, adopting behaviour that transgresses the norms and values of society. The first section of the chapter will therefore examine particular behaviour patterns observed among those residents who had been in prison, particularly those who had been in more than once, compared with those who had not been in prison. The Chi-square test showed a statistically significant relationship between prison admission and age. The ex-prisoner residents tended to come from the group aged 50 years and under (Table 9.1).

In describing these and other residents as 'subgroups', it is important to emphasize that the study found no strong evidence that men came into the hostels in groups. Thus, for example, there was no direct link between the hostels and the discharge policy from prisons, as may be

Table 9.1: Residents' (from both hostels) incidents of prison admission compared with residents' ages

Age	Prison admissions			
	None	1	1+	Total
Under 25 years	4	10	11	25
26–50 years	26	7	25	58
51–70 years	43	17	17	77
71 and over	11	3	3	17
Total	84	37	56	177

Chi-squared test, $p = <0.001$.

found in rehabilitation hostels. However, as will be exemplified, certain groupings of individuals demonstrated similar patterns of behaviour once they became residents.

Two distinct subgroups of the sample were recognized. There were a significantly higher number of impact of alcohol use events from among the ex-prisoner group than among the non-prisoner group. From the project nurse's detailed fieldwork observations, evidence emerged that a number of residents admitted being sent to prison for alcohol-related offences (Table 9.2).

Table 9.2: Residents' (from both hostels) incidents of prison admission compared with impact of alcohol events on residents' lives

	Prison admissions			
Impact of alcohol	None	1	1+	Total
Doesn't drink alcohol	15	7	12	34
No impact events	5	2	2	9
Some events	27	9	1	37
A number of events:				
may have an alcoholism problem	12	9	9	30
Considerable number of events:				
may have serious alcoholism problem	23	8	29	60
Total	82	35	53	170

Chi-squared test, $p = <0.001$.

Itinerant disorganized lifestyle

It is difficult, from the information gathered, to ascertain precisely any cause and effect relationship between alcohol misuse, prison admission and hostel residency, that is, whether drinking alcohol to excess was the starting point of the residents' lifestyle or whether living in hostels increased their alcohol consumption and criminal activity. However, a picture emerged of the ex-prisoner group of men. These residents tended to abuse alcohol, feel unwell, attend accident and emergency (A and E) departments and their general practitioner (GP) more frequently, display a high anxiety level and lead a chaotic lifestyle, sometimes getting banned from hostels for alcohol-related and/or violent behaviour. Several of these residents were found to be physically and psychologically fragile.

This scenario presents a familiar stereotype of homeless residents whose deviant, antisocial behaviour – recognized in Knight et al's

(1977) study of Borstal boys up to adulthood – cuts them off from society. A frequent use of A and E services, termed 'inappropriate' in some of the literature (Powell 1987a), was also seen. The ex-prisoner subgroup demonstrated a more frequent, chaotic use of the health-care services.

Some of the GPs, described in Chapter 6, stated how difficult it was for them to respond effectively when some residents attended their surgery under the influence of alcohol. In Chapter 5, a description was given of the project nurse receiving regular visits from some residents seeking help, although they were not in a position to respond to his advice or interventions because of their alcohol-related problems.

Challenges to the stereotypes: the non-prisoners

The number of times that a resident had been in prison proved a valid indicator for discovering a subgroup of men who tended to lead a chaotic lifestyle and were physically and psychologically vulnerable, often through their consumption of alcohol. However, 82 residents out of the 177 who answered had not been in prison, thus challenging the stereotype that all hostel residents were heavy-drinking ex-prisoners.

The majority (41 out of 53) of residents who had been in prison more than once had visited their GP within the previous 6 months. In Table 9.3, it can be seen that 34 of these ex-prisoner residents had attended A and E once or more within the past 2 years. The Chi-square test showed a significant difference in a comparison with residents who had not been in prison, who displayed a pattern of behaviour with less attendance at their GP and the A and E department. Two-thirds of the non-prisoners had not attended A and E in the previous 2 years.

Table 9.3: Residents' (from both hostels) incidents of prison admission compared with visits to accident and emergency in the past 2 years

| Visits to A&E in past 2 years | Prison admissions | | | |
	None	1	1+	Total
None	61	22	21	104
Once	12	7	11	30
Twice	6	5	4	15
More than twice	5	3	19	27
Total	84	37	55	176

Chi-squared test, p = <0.001.

However, the examination of attendance patterns of ex-prisoners at GPs and A and E (see Table 9.3), combined with the impact of alcohol use, demonstrated a statistically significant relationship for ex-prisoners and other residents who had alcohol-related problems with a more frequent use of health services. It has, however, also been shown that these residents are a distinct subgroup. A proportion of the residents display none of these behaviours.

Group values and norms

Change of aspirations

The analysis now moves to the experience and evidence of the effects of the hostels on the residents. The study found that residents demonstrated a varying degree of acclimatization, with concomitant lifestyle and attitude changes, that was connected with the length of time the resident had stayed in his hostel. These lifestyle and attitude changes demonstrated how some of the men identified with the hostel and other residents, and showed the formation of group values, norms and rationale for behaviour that differed from those of mainstream society.

In Table 9.4, for example, it may be seen that the longer a man stayed in a hostel, the more likely he was to call it 'home'. The relationship between these two variables was supported by the Chi-square test. It will also be seen that in the group of residents who had been in hostels for more than 6 years, 14 residents did not consider their hostel home. This was borne out by the author and project nurse's experience as they were often surprised at how some of the men had not acclimatized and accepted their hostel life as 'normal' or 'home' after a long period, whereas others accepted the life very quickly.

Table 9.4: Residents' (from both hostels) views of where 'home' was compared with the length of stay in their hostel

Length of stay	Where 'home' was			
	Here	With family	Elsewhere	Total
Under 1 year	21	41	17	79
1–5 years	19	18	16	53
6 years and over	29	7	7	43
Total	69	66	40	175

Chi-squared test, $p = <0.001$.

Table 9.5: Residents' (from both hostels) length of stay in their hostel compared with residents' ages

Age	Length of stay			
	Under 1 year	1–5 years	6 years and over	Total
Under 25 years	35	2	1	38
26–50 years	66	30	7	103
51–70 years	28	59	34	121
71 years and over	4	8	13	25
Total	133	99	55	287

Chi-squared test, $p = <0.001$.

As expected, the Chi-square test showed a significant difference between subgroups of residents (Table 9.5) when comparing the ages of the residents and their length of stay in the hostel. A large number of younger residents had lived in their hostel for under a year and were leading an unsettled transient lifestyle. Several of the older residents had lived in their hostel for longer. However, it is interesting to observe that 7 men in the 26–50 years age group had been in their hostel for 6 years or over, demonstrating how a few men had become long-stay residents at a younger age. Also noteworthy was that almost half of the 71 years and over age group (who might have been expected to be long-term residents) had in fact been residents for 5 years or less. Thus whereas a resident's age may be a useful general indicator to distinguish between long-term and short-term residency, Table 9.5 demonstrates that this is not always the case.

What became apparent was that a number of residents throughout the age range (including 12 residents who were 71 or over) had come into hostel accommodation within the previous 5 years. The four residents of 71 and over who had been resident for under 1 year were in the Main Study Hostel, four from each hostel comprising the men who had been resident for 1–5 years.

A closer examination revealed that these admissions had often resulted from a breakdown in health, the loss of the significant woman in their life (this perhaps supporting the 'transition' theory of formative life events affecting the individual, which was cited earlier) and an increasing inability to cope. For this group of residents, the hostels were a bizarre alternative to sheltered housing or eventide homes. The hostels thus provided accommodation to residents with a wide range of social and health-care needs.

In summary, Table 9.4 above demonstrates important findings. The majority of residents whose length of stay was under 1 year saw home as being with their family. This perception declined in the residents who had been resident between 1 and 5 years and very substantially declined for those who had been resident for 6 years and over. It should be noted that the sharpest decline in the perception of the hostel as home appears to be between the shorter-term (under 1 year) and the medium-term (between 1 and 5 years) residents. In terms of implications for the nursing assessment and for the regular monitoring of hostel residents, these findings may assist nurses as they respond to the differing needs of individuals who have recently become resident in a hostel and those, longer-term, residents who have established themselves in their hostel.

Having demonstrated that the reasons men gave for becoming residents were sometimes complex, it can be shown that difficulties were encountered by residents of all ages and with all lengths of stay. The analysis now moves to a presentation of the difficulties that some residents experienced and the negative adaptations they sometimes made towards the project nurse's interventions.

Conflict and co-operation

This section of the chapter examines some of the qualitative evidence of the study that describes examples of the residents' positive and negative interactions with the project nurse, the GPs and other health professionals. Its purpose is to exemplify more specific interactions, give examples of individual men and provide a more detailed profile of the residents' experience than can be offered by the statistical data. The qualitative data are taken from the systematic observation and recording in the incident diary and residents' notes by the project nurse, and from the formation of themes and paradigms described in Chapters 3 and 5.

Conflict: negative patterns of interaction with health professionals

Reluctance to attend GP

The project nurse, in his assessments, discovered some of the residents' views regarding access to their GP when he offered to refer the resident to his doctor. Fifteen men told the project nurse that the GP was too far away and 27 that they were reluctant to attend. The reasons for a reluctance to attend varied from disinclination to follow up their health assessment, to a more focused apprehension such as previous bad experiences with health centre personnel or embarrassment at attending their GP. With help, many of these residents overcame their reluctance.

Residents passing responsibility to the project nurse

Fourteen residents were generally happy for the project nurse to help them but were unwilling to co-operate actively. They would, for example, ask the project nurse to make appointments or write letters and follow them up. One man wanted to go into a centre for his alcohol problem, but only if the project nurse organized everything. What is interesting about these 14 residents and their views is that the author was told by several of the health professionals he interviewed that this attitude predominated among homeless men. Although this is a significant group (out of the total number of 66), it is by no means a majority. The 'handing over' of responsibility to others will be revisited later in this chapter.

Attendance at the GP for a sickness certificate

Five residents told the project nurse that they were attending their doctor for a sickness benefit certificate but did not use the opportunity to tell the doctor about new problems. Although this is a small number, the study found that there were other men, who did not require intervention at the time of the study but who were interviewed in both hostels, who regularly attended their GPs without informing them of existing problems.

'Antisocial' behaviour: negative interactions

Some of the difficulties that the project nurse encountered in carrying out the study were more directly confrontational reactions to himself and to the study. Twenty-one residents were recorded as treating the project nurse with open suspicion, six of them exhibiting aggressive behaviour. Nineteen residents directly refused to take part in the study when asked, and another four residents refused to complete the assessment interview. Seventeen residents failed to attend appointments made for them.

Much of the behaviour displayed to the project nurse in these occurrences could be classed as antisocial and threatening. The project nurse's role was to work with these residents, so he persevered with them. He kept contact with the residents during the study by engaging them in conversation and by making his presence known in the sitting room so that they had opportunities to approach him as often as they wished.

It is, however, interesting to compare the project nurse's approach to one of the district nurse's comments described in Chapter 6. She stated that 'her GP' did not like female nurses to go into hostels, although another said that violence was 'not usually a problem'. This possible gender issue will be discussed in Chapter 10.

The implications for practice are interesting. First, these reactions demonstrate that health professionals define 'no go' areas, particularly when faced with antisocial behaviour, although there is no evidence to show that professionals are any more at risk in hostels, for example, than anywhere else. Second, there is a suggestion from the professional responses that potential patients' behaviour has to correspond to their own values before they are deemed suitable for care. This point will be revisited in Chapter 10.

Summary of analysis of negative interaction with health professionals

The behaviour patterns demonstrated by the men in both hostels, and by a closer examination of the behaviour of residents in the Main Study Hostel, yielded some insights. The use of A and E services by men in the Main Study Hostel was particularly marked and different from that of the men in the Comparison Hostel. The Main Study Hostel was nearer the hospital than was the Comparison Hostel, but the difference is nonetheless significant. Two-thirds of the residents in the Comparison Hostel had not been to A and E in the previous 2 years. A much higher proportion of the residents in the Main Study Hostel came into the vulnerable, alcohol problem, ex-prisoner, high-morbidity group.

Co-operation: residents displaying complex, positive interactions with health professionals

The exposition of negative factors such as the 'inappropriate' use of health services and difficult interactions experienced by the project nurse has been important. In order to present a more complete description, it is also important to demonstrate some of the complexity of the mutual interactions between the men, the hostel staff and the project nurse.

Presented below is a case study highlighting the positive side, the companionship and the demonstration of humanity also referred to in the previous chapter with regard to the interdependence and self-concept modes.

I.T. was a 51-year-old man who was in many ways atypical of the hostel-dweller. He was well dressed, well groomed and articulate. He did not drink alcohol and held a professional qualification (teacher). Before taking up residence in the hostel, he had spent a number of years living in Spain with friends and only returned because of financial difficulties. However, below the surface, there were common factors that he shared with many other residents: he had in the past been treated for alcoholism, which led to the loss of his teaching post, he was divorced from his wife and he had lost contact with his two daughters. He had taken on the role of carer for another resident. Every morning and evening, he looked after A. by cleaning his right eye socket. This task used to be carried out by a district nurse, who now visits monthly in a supervisory capacity.

This interaction is representative of the large number of cases of 'looking out for' other residents that the study witnessed, often not for any discernible material benefit to the individual giving the assistance.

Among other activities that were recorded as taking place between the men, the staff and the study, were 17 men who had regular contact with health and social services. These residents were already involved in relationships with these services. These had been facilitated, in the main, by the hostel staff as the primary referral agents, although some of the residents had instigated the action themselves. The project nurse also recorded 10 occasions on which the hostel staff referred men with health needs to him. When the study started, the hostel staff continued as referrers as well as acting as effective go-betweens for many of the residents who were often reluctant to approach a stranger.

Companionship

Part of the complex interpersonal interactions described above may be illustrated as in Tables 9.6 and 9.7. The Chi-square test demonstrated a significant relationship between the length of time the men had lived in their hostel and those with whom they wished to live (Table 9.6). There was also a tendency to prefer to live with friends and others as the men became older (Table 9.7). As has been described, residents' attitudes towards their accommodation tended to change the longer they were resident and the older they were. They also developed an affinity for the company of the friends they had made among other residents and, if given the choice, would prefer to live in accommodation with them.

Internal barriers: individuals' perceptions of the hostel

Rootedness and uprootedness

It is interesting to note how few young residents wished to live with friends or other residents, perhaps reflecting a more transient unstable

Table 9.6: Residents' view of whom they would like to live with compared with length of stay in their hostel

| Length of stay in hostel | Companionship preference | | | |
	Wife/partner	Friends	Alone	Total
Under 1 year	27	9	41	77
1–5 years	6	25	20	51
6 years and over	6	25	14	41
Total	37	57	75	169

Chi-squared test, p = <0.001.

Table 9.7: Residents' view of whom they would like to live with compared with residents' ages

| Age | Companionship preference | | | |
	Wife/partner	Friends	Alone	Total
Under 25 years	13	1	11	25
26–50 years	14	9	32	55
51–70 years	11	32	31	74
71 years and over	0	15	3	18
Total	38	57	77	172

Chi-squared test, p = <0.001.

outlook and lifestyle (the 'uprootedness' described earlier), but that this became the more popular option among older men. However, some men, given the choice, would always wish to live alone. There was evidence of the men tending to become more 'rooted' with the length of stay in the hostels and loss of contact with family. This may be interpreted as a recognition of the significance and shared values of 'place', that is, the hostel.

A structured, controlled environment

Two distinct groups have emerged: those who, because of some disruption in their life, seek or end up in hostel accommodation, and those who make a lifestyle choice, seeing the hostel as being a positive advantage. The time spent living in the hostels has an effect, as many men move from the first group into the second. Many of the second, more rooted, group were witnessed by the project nurse and the author as having more complex networks and interactions with friends among other residents and elsewhere, although the study did not find evidence that these men actually chose their hostels because specific friends were already resident there.

Some residents never made the transition to rootedness and always preferred to be somewhere else, no matter how long they were resident. As with the ex-prisoner' group, no evidence was found that any residents in the more rooted group had come into the hostels in groups; the companionship, interactions and lifestyle appeared to emanate from the time of their hostel residency.

Functionalism

Why the hostels are there

Another aspect of deviancy theory – functionalism – considers institutions and social phenomena that appear to be entirely negative and/or detrimental but provide a functional, if negative, role integral to the efficient working of the society. The example often cited is prostitution, as a social need rather than a market force. Great care has to be taken when considering the sometimes negative role of hostels and the residents' way of life. The author is neither labelling nor stigmatizing the residents, nor is he making judgements about them. However, the author recognized phenomena in his study of the particular social environment of the hostels that appeared to demonstrate particular rules, customs, values and routines. What follows is a presentation of the exploration of this social and interactional setting that attempts to provide an analytical framework in order to gain some understanding – to 'make sense' of the phenomena seen.

The need for simple safe accommodation

There appeared to be a need on the part of the residents for the provision of relatively safe, simple accommodation. An example of this need was demonstrated by J.B., who, although not typical in other ways, exemplified the need for uncomplicated, low-level housing. J.B. appears to have found a way of coping by using the hostel rather than other alternatives.

J.B. was a 50-year-old man who entered homeless accommodation after becoming unemployed, turning to excessive alcohol use and eventually breaking up with his wife. At the time of interview, he was attending a College of Further Education 2 days per week studying photography. In addition to this, he was about to start on a government Employment Creation Scheme, which would again further his interest in photography. He demonstrated a further commitment to his chosen career when he told me that he was paying off the equipment that he was currently using; this hire-purchase agreement had become necessary when his camera and other equipment were stolen from his room. To achieve these aims, J.B. found that the simple hostel life assisted him to cope. He did not have to worry about domestic complications, and although he did recognize the unpleasant side of hostel living, it suited him until he could get his 'head together'.

Residents moving from other hostels to the Main Study Hostel

As has been described, the two study hostels were different in a number of ways. Chief among these differences were the condition of the buildings and the facilities provided. The project nurse also found that many of the residents in the Main Study Hostel had been banned from other hostels. Table 9.8 demonstrates the number of residents who had lived in other hostels before arriving at the Main Study Hostel. The hostel staff stated that they regularly admitted residents who had been banned from Council hostels.

In the Comparison Hostel, there were also a number of residents who had come from other hostels. The Comparison Hostel was the District Council's admissions hostel, in which residents who were coming into, or returning to, the hostel system were admitted. These residents had sometimes been in prison or had had alternating periods of living in hostels and living at home. Residents banned from other Council hostels were not admitted to the Comparison Hostel.

Table 9.8: Residents' (from the Main Study Hostel) length of stay in homeless accomodation compared with the length of stay in their present hostel

Length of stay in this hostel	Length of stay in homeless accommodation			
	Under 1 year	1–5 years	6 years and over	Total
Under 1 year	14	8	15	37
1–5 years	1	17	9	27
6 years and over	0	1	19	20
Total	15	26	43	84

Chi-squared test, p = <0.001.

'Sump' factor: negative rationale for Main Study Hostel's existence

The combination of high vulnerability and disorganized patterns of service use, described earlier, including what might be considered antisocial behaviour, combined with the evidence of residents being banned from other hostels, may support the hypothesis that there is a need for the Main Study Hostel as a functional, if negative, necessity. The expression 'sump' was used by some professionals when referring to the Main Study Hostel.

Continuing this line of argument, it would appear that the Main Study Hostel had an important functional role acting as a buffer between banned hostel residents and the street. This enabled two circumstances to prevail. First, it meant that there was somewhere for residents to go when they were unwelcome elsewhere. Second, it might be said that other hostels could afford to have 'higher' or stricter standards of residency in the knowledge that if they did have to evict a resident, he would not have to sleep on the street.

This is not the place for conspiracy theories, but it is interesting to note that despite occasional strong protests from public, political and other sources regarding the condition of the Main Study Hostel, it has not been closed down. After the fire, which happened during the course of the study, and in which one young resident died, there was consideration of this point. The main reaction, expressed to the author and project nurse by hostel staff and others working in the homeless accommodation field, was the question of where all the men would be placed.

Table 9.8 above shows that 32 residents had lived in other hostels before arriving in the Main Study Hostel. It should be noted that 15 of the residents who had stayed in the Main Study Hostel for less than 1 year had been in hostel accommodation for 6 or more years. Thirty-three residents had lived in other hostels before reaching the Comparison Hostel (Table 9.9). Five residents who had stayed in the Comparison Hostel for under 1 year had been in hostel accommodation for 6 or more years.

The apparent need for the Main Study Hostel as a 'sump' or 'buffer' is important. It can be seen that the Main Study Hostel in particular has a pragmatic, functional role as a method of controlling a potential problem that may provoke protest from either the public or the public service agencies, that is, the problem of a large number of homeless men, possibly sleeping rough, visible on the streets. The advantage of the Main Study Hostel may be that of taking men off the streets so that they will make less demand on other services, for example housing.

Table 9.9: Residents' (from the Comparison Hostel) length of stay in homeless accomodation compared with the length of stay in their present hostel

Length of stay in this hostel	Length of stay in homeless accommodation			
	Under 1 year	1–5 years	6 years and over	Total
Under 1 year	27	12	5	44
1–5 years	0	12	16	28
6 years and over	0	0	24	24
Total	27	24	45	96

Chi-squared test, $p = <0.001$.

Taking this point further, the Main Study Hostel contains the men, relieving the housing and other services of a large presence who might otherwise deter other potential users of these services from using them. Judged from this perspective, the advantage of the hostel might be that it separates out a particularly problematic group of individuals.

These points have been suggested by some of the evidence in the study, particularly by the movement of residents into the Main Study Hostel from other hostels and by the fact that, despite years of neglect and reports of its potential closure, the Main Study Hostel continues to exist and provide accommodation. The next section examines some of the evidence that provided an insight into what the residents wanted from the hostels.

The group's needs: the hostel as an institution

The passive administrative domestic role

One of the important advantages of taking a sociological perspective, which was supported by the author's experience during the study, was that by studying the actions of the group, an idea was gained into why they were pursuing their present lifestyle. For example, by interviewing the men, a possible rationale behind the choice to live in hostel-type accommodation was discovered. This rationale counterbalances the views of some health professionals and others who may regard the group as behaving in an aberrant or deviant manner simply because the residents are not doing what is 'normal'.

As highlighted in the introduction to this chapter, the author and project nurse's professional training and attitudes before the study tended towards the examination and treatment of the residents as individuals. No particular emphasis was be placed on how or why the 'patient' was there; the important point was to accept that he was there and to proceed with the assessment and treatment. Looking at the residents as a group held connotations of stereotyping. On closer examination, however, considering the rationale proved useful, with practical benefits.

Specifically, the study found that there were many residents who wished to live in hostel-type accommodation. For these residents, problems arose from their personal state of health, their financial circumstances and the conditions within the particular hostel. These residents preferred to live in hostel accommodation as it enabled them to adopt a passive domestic administrative role, that is, they preferred to hand over the responsibility of providing a warm, dry, lit home, with a bed, to another agency. By paying their board and lodging, and living in a hostel, these residents were able to live in this minimalist role.

The need for accommodation to provide for the passive role may be seen in other groups of people, particularly men: the Civil Service, for example, provides hostel accommodation for its employees. Even when living at home, many of the residents in the study told the project nurse and author that they tended to leave the active domestic administrative role to someone else, mainly the significant woman of the home. Hostels, therefore, provide a useful service, and many of the men, particularly in the Comparison Hostel (with its better facilities), were found to live there from choice, enjoying the companionship. Residents would, however, as seen above, arrive in the Main Study Hostel, with its disreputable reputation, for a variety of reasons, many coming from other hostels, some following misbehaviour and banishment.

Other factors influencing men becoming residents

Another group of residents had arrived in hostel accommodation owing to some dysfunction in their home, health or financial circumstances. In the Main Study Hostel, J.V. was an example of a man whose change in circumstances resulted in his arriving at the hostel and adopting the passive domestic administrative role.

J.V. was a 38-year-old man who had recently taken up residence in the hostel. He was atypical in so far as his use of this type of homeless accommodation was different from that of residents of a similar age, and he was generally in employment, having become unemployed only a few months prior to moving into the hostel. He is a pipe fitter/welder to trade and tends to work on short-term contracts, moving around the country to find work. While in employment, he generally lives in rented or bed and breakfast accommodation and has therefore not settled down in one area for any length of time. He differs from those of a similar age as he does not have a history of living in hostels, and in this respect is more like the younger hostel-dwellers (less than 25 years of age); however, unlike this group, he does have a regular if fragmented employment history. Prior to taking up residence in the hostel, he was living with his mother and sister, but had an argument with his sister and left the family home.

This 'passive' choice of living resonates some of the deviancy theory debate. Kitsuse (in Spitzer and Denzin 1968, p 41) describes how some forms of behaviour, whilst 'institutionally permitted', are considered deviant because the behaviour 'clearly represents a departure from the cultural model in which residents are obliged to move onward and upward in the social hierarchy'. The concept of choosing a style of life that is 'institutionally permitted' (the hostels), but rejecting the 'cultural model' of social mobility by choosing the passive domestic role, not only exists in theory, but has also been demonstrated, it is suggested, by the evidence in this study as well as in reality. The 'departure' from normal models is also suggested by the practice of calling hostels 'homeless accommodation' when there is clearly some evidence that men are choosing the hostels as their home.

Attitudes of professionals and others towards the group

Are the residents 'homeless'?

As discussed earlier, some of the residents came to the hostel and, either immediately or after a period of time, considered the hostel to be home or the centre of their existence and lifestyle. Others considered their residency in the hostel to be an aberration that put them outside what they considered their chosen life. These residents were sometimes clear in their own minds about what had caused this – alcohol, a domestic rift, unemployment or bad health, for example. Some residents did not accept the hostel as the centre of their life no matter how long they stayed there. This may be seen in Table 9.10. Whereas 48 residents who had been resident for 6 years or more considered their hostel to be home, 43 still thought home to be with their families or elsewhere.

The residents' feelings of where their home was and the differences between residents emphasizes an important point. Although, for administrative, professional and political purposes, hostel accommodation is officially called 'homeless accommodation', this does not take

Table 9.10: Views of residents (from both hostels) on where home was compared with the last time the residents had lived with their families

Last time with their family	Where the home is			
	Here	With family	Elsewhere	Total
Under 1 year	4	18	7	29
1–5 years	13	21	13	47
6 years and over	48	25	18	91
Not lived with family	2	1	0	3
Total	67	65	38	170

Chi-squared test, $p = <0.001$.

into account the complexity of the men's attitudes to their position – one man in the Pilot Study Hostel had tried to buy his room from the Council under the government 'right-to-buy' provision. The importance of this point becomes clear when trying to provide health and social care for hostel residents, taking into account their attitudes and expectations. This will be discussed in detail in Chapter 10.

Professional attitudes

Even health personnel whose attitude was positive towards the residents – wanting to help and provide the best care – appeared to consider the residents different because they did not express themselves assertively or seek to 'better themselves'. The evidence of the expert panel showed that although the the panel was in broad agreement with the actions and procedures undertaken by the district nurses who received referrals, those district nurses had taken only a minimalist first aid or rescue role with the residents.

The district nurses dealt efficiently with the problem with which they were presented, but they did not necessarily provide the breadth of mainstream service exemplified by the expert panel. This suggests that the residents were considered by the district nurses not to require the same level of service as others. For example, one of the expert panel described how she would assist one of the elderly residents:

He's much better off in a nursing home than he had been in this hostel. If I was really to assess him, I would examine what his mobility was like, what treatment he was having for his arthritis and his oedema, whether he'd ever been seen by a rheumatologist, what his dietary habits were, what his fluid intake and output were, whether he had any physiotherapy, how much exercise he was able to do, how much of his time he spent in fresh air, how much time he spent just sitting around. This assessment would provide a firm basis for referral.

The district nurse who received the referral confined herself to assessment and monitoring within the hostel.

As mentioned earlier, it is possible that professional attitudes include the view that individuals must achieve a certain standard before they are deemed worthy of service. Those who do not achieve this standard are served only by a minimal service or are not given any service at all.

> The dedicated pursuit of culturally approved goals, the adherence to normatively sanctioned means – these imply a certain self-restraint, effort, discipline, inhibition. What is the effect of others who, though their activities do not manifestly damage our own interests, are morally undisciplined, who give themselves up to idleness, self indulgence, or forbidden vices? What effect does the propinquity of the wicked have upon the peace of mind of the virtuous? (Cohen in Rock and McIntosh 1974, p 236)

In his discussion of deviancy, drugs and the media, Young (in Rock and McIntosh1974) uses this quotation to express the concept of 'moral indignation'. The quotation is apt, because it demonstrates fundamental assumptions made by many of the health professionals when referrals were made to them. They appeared to see their role more as giving minimal first aid and/or rescue from the worst effects of ill-health than as making available what could be described as normal provision.

These assumptions were, in the main, not expressed in a morally judgemental way. One GP talked about expectations for this 'class' of person, but he was unusual. However, the project nurse, having completed his assessment, would sometimes find it difficult to obtain treatment for a resident. The source of this difficulty centred around the attitude that the professional would not make an overtly 'old-fashioned', moralistic analysis of the resident's situation (described in the quotation), apportioning blame, implying the need for punishment or expressing the view that he did not deserve to have treatment. The analysis and rationale for little or no intervention, presented to the author by many of the health professionals he interviewed, could be paraphrased thus:

Given that many of these residents have chosen to eschew a more regular, restrained way of life, they are going to end up in trouble. They live in bad conditions and lead an unhealthy lifestyle. It is, therefore, not surprising that they are depressed, anxious or suffering from physical illness. Treatment may be expected to be of limited use.

This pragmatic, if fatalistic view, may sound more 'professional' and is less derogatory than a judgemental, punitive view that the men deserve their conditions and minimal service because of their behaviour. In practical terms, however, this fatalistic professional view appeared to have the same effect as the more moralistic standpoint. The fatalistic view also contradicted the experience of the project nurse. In the previous chapter, the residents' positive response to the project nurse, the study and the health services was described. It would be wrong to claim that all the residents responded positively to intervention: indeed, many residents avoided the study. However, positive reactions to help were displayed by some individuals.

Similarities with other marginalized groups

The attitudes outlined above were also described in much of the literature described in Chapter 2 regarding other marginalized groups, particularly individuals being ostracized and the adverse effects of regulation. Similarities could be seen by the project nurse and author between the treatment of the mentally ill from ethnic minorities, who were often treated as criminals (Medical Campaign Project and Campaign for Homeless and Rootless 1991) and the hostel residents. In addition, the physical condition of the Main Study Hostel, despite regulation, was poor and often detrimental to the well-being of residents, particularly the frail elderly. This mirrored descriptions in the literature and the author's professional experience of prisons (CIBA Foundation 1973)

A basic right in Britain and elsewhere is that an individual can approach, or refuse, health services as he or she sees fit. The effect is that most services depend on the individual seeking out help, so the service is mainly reactive. Exceptions to this are child surveillance and vaccination programmes, but even here responsibility lies with the consumer or parent (Rappaport 1981, Drennan and Stearn 1986). This service approach tends to assume that individuals who do not approach the service do not want it. Thus, attitudes to proactive work by professionals and government may be mixed. If a marginalized person 'chooses' not to claim benefits, a common example, what is the role of the service in a consumer-led society? (McDonald 1986).

Implications of professional attitudes for practice

The recognition of the passive role taken by some of the men and the 'handing over' of areas of social and domestic responsibility to others has important implications for the delivery of appropriate health and nursing services to these men. Their lack of assertiveness, and perhaps assumptions about this attitude made by health professionals with whom they come into contact, may lead to misunderstanding and cause health professionals to see the men's health problems as discrete items to be addressed reactively, that is, only as they are presented by the individual rather than as an holistic set of health-care needs to be proactively identified and acted upon by the health professional.

This study has recognized both the reactive role, demonstrated by the district nurses and described in Chapter 6, and the proactive role, demonstrated by the project nurse and described in Chapter 5. The analysis in this chapter has perhaps highlighted that these two approaches are not two ends of a spectrum but instead demonstrate a fundamental difference in philosophical outlook on the part of health professionals, particularly nurses, regarding their duties and obligations in the context of caring for homeless and other marginalized people.

On the one hand, nurses and other professionals are encouraged to 'empower' patients to assert their needs, take control of their lives and make specific demands to appropriate agencies as 'consumers', to which the nurse reacts with specialist skills. On the other, it may be seen that some individuals do not want, or are unable, to adopt an assertive role, in which case the nurse's role is to seek and respond to often unexpressed need.

Conclusion: challenging the stereotypes

The use of deviancy theory and the sociological device of examining the residents and their behaviour for rationale and group traits has provided illuminating insights. This 'lens' has demonstrated that whereas stereotypes, particularly those associated with alcohol abuse and criminality, depicted in the literature and described by professionals to the author and project nurse may apply to some of the men, they cannot be applied across the whole group.

A subgroup of residents appear to live in the hostels as a transient period in an 'uprooted', violent and unhealthy life. Other residents, having arrived in hostel accommodation (for a variety of reasons) are attempting to find 'rootedness', choice and a reasonable interaction with the world. Some of these men seek accommodation that enables them to take a passive role with regard to providing a home and prefer the companionship of fellow residents.

A number of differential indicators have been suggested that may assist professionals, particularly nurses, to identify individuals within the two main subgroups, that is, those individuals who are uprooted, transient and homeless, and those who may be more rooted and have made a positive choice to stay in hostel accommodation. These differential indicators include a history of prison, the extent of use of the health services, anxiety level and the answers to such simple questions as 'How do you feel?' and 'Where is home?' The next chapter will discuss the practical use of this knowledge.

Chapter 10
Discussion and recommendations

The purpose of this chapter is to bring together the different strands of the study and analysis by presenting a summary and discussion of the findings. This will be followed by recommendations for practice and future research.

Important overall findings

It is important at this point to highlight four points discovered during the study that will, with the benefit of hindsight, change my approach to undertaking a similar study in the future. By stating them here, I hope to create a clear context in which the more specific findings may be seen.

Constraints

In the preparation for the study, certain elements of practice in the proposed study were not obvious. This constrained, to a certain extent, the scope of the study. These constraints were time, access and a lack of previous similar work. It was not known how stable the population of single homeless men was, whether a large proportion would be willing to engage with the study and how much time they would be prepared to spend in the interviews. These factors combined meant that the study and approach were pioneering in nature. As it happened, the population, particularly in the Main Study Hostel, was very stable, the majority were willing to engage in the study and, once recruited, they were (with a few notable exceptions) extremely obliging in terms of time.

Had this been known before the study commenced, it might have been possible to use more complex validated tools, particularly in relation to physical and social function. It might also have been possible to introduce into the design follow-up interviews providing a more precise insight into clinical and personal outcomes. Previous

213

work in the area had suggested a more transient population (Atkinson 1987, Featherstone and Ashmore 1988, Williams and Allen 1989).

Critique of the validated tools

Barthel Index

Taking into account the constraints, it was decided to use a simple tool to define physical function, one which was, as far as possible, neither environment nor context specific (to ensure that the men's homeless state did not distort the findings). The Barthel Index (Mahoney and Barthel 1965) measures only physical function and therefore appeared to have the simplicity required for this study. However, as the findings demonstrate, the outcome of its use was not as predicted.

First, the Barthel Index is more successfully used on a recognizable physically disabled population to discern levels of relative normal and abnormal function (originally being used with patients who had suffered a stroke). Most people in the general population score very highly, and it is limited in detecting disability or functional problems if the individual is able to achieve the tasks by himself or if he tolerates a certain amount of dysfunction (taking 20 minutes to get to the toilet or urinary dribbling, for example).

Second, the tool and the disability themselves are entirely environment/context dependent. One is disabled because one cannot achieve certain tasks in particular circumstances, which therefore dictates where one can live, work and exist. Because the Comparison Hostel had better facilities, it was possible for disabled people to live there. The population scores on the Barthel Index thus described the context better than they described the individuals.

Taking the previous points together with the fact that the men usually demonstrated a willingness to spend time with the study, it may be possible in future studies to use more complex tools examining function and quality of life, taking particular care to exclude or adapt questions that would obviously provide ambivalent answers given the homeless context (such as questions regarding holidays, possessions and activities).

Hospital Anxiety and Depression Scale

Conversely, the use of the HAD Scale proved immensely valuable even though it too had been chosen, in part, for its simplicity, ease and speed of use. The Present State Examination (PSE) (Win et al 1974), which was considered, would not have been appropriate (even in hindsight) as, even with the men's co-operation, it would have taken too long (1.5

hours) and the PSE concentrates on psychotic illness, which would not have discovered this study's major findings regarding anxiety and possible biogenic depression. There is also some question over whether the PSE could be administered by any community nurse as a primary assessment tool.

Limitations of the study

Taking the constraints and the critique of the Barthel Index into account, it is essential to stress that this study considered only one hostel in one city. Comparative elements were included, in particular the Comparison Hostel and the provision of background context in the literature review. The study does not therefore claim that the men in the study are representative of homeless men in Britain, for example, although other workers in the area may see a resonance with their own experience in this study.

Use of the district nurse: impact on the findings

As described in Chapter 1, I came from a district nursing background and was motivated to initiate a rigorous study arising from exploratory work undertaken in the area of homelessness as a practising district nurse. For the purposes of an academic study, it was also necessary to be as precise as possible when describing and setting up the study. However, as an individual, and, as is supported by the findings, I do not categorize nurses into tight professional bands, classing myself only as a community nurse. In terms of practice, what is more important is the clinical competency of the individual nurse and the ability/autonomy to proactively case-find, assess and monitor the physical and psychological well-being of individuals in a defined group.

A community psychiatric nurse attached to a psychiatrist's caseload in a hospital who had little experience of treating physical illness would have difficulty in undertaking the work described in this study. However, many community nurses now work across professional boundaries, and it is suggested that the findings of this study are not specific to the district nurse but instead identify a model of community nursing practice.

Summary of specific findings

Differences between hostels

In Chapter 4, statistically significant differences between the two hostels' (Main Study Hostel and Comparison Hostel) sample groups were demonstrated. The demographic profile varied in relation to, for example, the length of time the residents had stayed in the hostel. Differences were also found between the hostel facilities. These differences, while interesting, did not, however, impinge on the main purpose of this study, namely the description and evaluation of district nursing intervention. They therefore do not feature highly in the discussion or recommendations in this chapter.

The main aim of the study was to assess the health and nursing needs of a group of homeless men and to evaluate a system of referral and of district nursing intervention designed to meet the needs identified. This aim was achieved successfully, and a variety of important information and insights were discovered.

The sample: data collection

Two forms of data were collected: quantitative and qualitative. The quantitative data were collected by the project nurse in the Main Study Hostel, and the author in the Comparison Hostel. The qualitative data were collected by the project nurse only in the Main Study Hostel. The quantitative data will be addressed first.

Main Study Hostel

Data, for example age and length of stay, were obtained on all 168 residents. Of these residents, 106 were approached for assessment interviews by the project nurse. These 106 men formed the sample.

Comparison Hostel

Some data were obtained on all 227 residents (for some only their name and age being available). Of these men, 180 were approached for interviews by the researcher. One hundred men participated in interviews.

Study results

Results from the questionnaire and validated tools were analysed using the Statistical Package for the Social Sciences (1990).

Age and length of stay in the hostel

The largest group of men in each hostel were aged between 51 and 70 years (50% in the Main Study Hostel and 53% in the Comparison Hostel). There were more young men (under 25 years old) in the Comparison Hostel, which was used as an emergency admission unit by Glasgow District Council.

Two broad groups of men emerged in both hostels, although not every resident was typical of either group:

- Group 1 tended to be older and had made a choice to live in hostel-type accommodation with other residents. Many of them considered the hostel to be their home. This group had a lower prison record and often a lower anxiety level.
- Group 2 tended to be younger and had come to live in a hostel because of some breakdown in their family relationships, social circumstances or health. Alcohol use, a high anxiety level and higher prison admittance were seen in this group. This group tended to think of the hostel not as their home but as a temporary alternative.

Marital status

Half of the sample in both hostels were single, and approximately a third were divorced or separated. Twelve of the men in the Main Study Hostel were widowers, as were six in the Comparison Hostel.

Employment

Of those interviewed in the Main Study Hostel, only 4 men were in employment, and of those interviewed in the Comparison Hostel only 2. These men informed both the project nurse and the author that having to give the hostel as their address had a detrimental effect on their chance of employment. Of all the men interviewed from both hostels, just over half had not been in employment for 6 years or more.

Registration with a general practitioner

Eighty-six per cent of the men in the Main Study Hostel and 95% of those in the Comparison Hostel were currently registered with a general practitioner (GP). Over half of the respondents in both the Main Study Hostel and the Comparison Hostel lived within 1 mile of their GP's surgery.

In the Main Study Hostel, 41% were currently receiving treatment from their GP, as were 49% in the Comparison Hostel. In most cases, treatment was for physical illness. Over 55% of the men in both hostels had visited their GP within the past 3 months, in many cases to collect repeat prescriptions and/or sickness certificates.

Hospital admissions

Within the previous 2 years, half of the men in both hostels had been hospital inpatients, predominantly as a result of diagnosed physical illness. Only 10% of men in both hostels had never been in hospital.

Twenty-one per cent of the Main Study Hostel sample and 14% of the Comparison Hostel sample had been admitted to a mental hospital within the past 5 years. There was little evidence that men had been discharged from long-stay care directly into hostel accommodation. It was, however, obvious that some had been in long-term care, had been discharged into supervised accommodation and at a later date had become hostel residents following a breakdown in their social circumstances.

Nursing visits

Nine men in the Main Study Hostel had been visited by a nurse, 4 by a district nurse and 5 by a community psychiatric nurse (CPN). Seven men had received nursing visits in the Comparison Hostel, 3 from district nurses and 4 from CPNs. District nurses only visited following a referral from a GP or hospital. The Greater Glasgow Health Board specialist CPN team for the homeless had started working in the hostels in 1992 and was building up its caseload. This will be discussed later.

Use of the accident and emergency department

There was a considerable difference in the pattern of visits to the accident and emergency (A and E) Department (at the Glasgow Royal Infirmary) between the two samples. Under half of the Main Study Hostel sample had not attended an A and E department within the previous 2 years, compared with two-thirds of those in the Comparison Hostel. A third of the Main Study Hostel sample had attended twice or more, compared with 13% of the Comparison Hostel sample. It should be stated that the Main Study Hostel is sited nearer to the hospital than is the Comparison Hostel.

Despite these geographical considerations, the difference between the patterns of use of the A and E department is significant, these patterns appearing to be related both to the residents' subjective view of their state of health and to the frequency of their admission to hospital. There was also a positive relationship between a high A and E department use, a prison record and a high impact of alcohol on lifestyle.

Prison record

Half of both the Main Study Hostel and the Comparison Hostel sample had been in prison. Thirty-eight per cent of the men in the Main Study sample had been a prisoner on more than two occasions. Many of the men in each hostel went to prison on a regular basis, often for alcohol-related offences. This may account for the high anxiety level recorded in this group (a positive correlation between alcohol use and high anxiety level being recognized in the literature), the number of visits to their doctor and to A and E, and how they felt about their state of health.

Residents' perception of their state of health

The question 'How do you feel?' proved one of the most useful questions in the study. Just over half of the sample in the Main Study Hostel and two-thirds of the Comparison Hostel sample said that they felt well. Significant statistical relationships were found between those men who stated that they felt unwell or ill, with several hospital admissions, raised levels of anxiety and depression, a high use of the A and E department and an increased impact of alcohol use on lifestyle.

Preferences for companionship and type of accommodation

Similarly, asking residents, 'Where would you like to live?', 'With whom would you like to live?' and 'Where is home?' provided great insight into residents' present well-being, aspirations and adaptive processes.

Two-thirds of the sample in the Main Study Hostel and the Comparison sample wanted to live in a house or flat, but a third of the men wanted to live in hostel accommodation. Although the largest group in the Main Study Hostel wanted to live alone, a third wanted to live with their wife and/or family. This evidence, borne out by the project nurse's experience, showed that residents' personal aspirations had an effect on how they felt at the present and on their level of contentment with their circumstances and adaptation. The project nurse found men who had lived in hostels for many years but who wanted to live with their families and tended to see their lifestyle as aberrant or dysfunctional because of this. Conversely, other men who had lived in hostels only a short time seemed to be reasonably happy with their lot and considered themselves to be living a 'normal' lifestyle.

Physical function – the Barthel Index

The Barthel Index, which scores physical function from 0 (low) to 100 (high), showed differences between the hostels. Ninety per cent of the men in the Main Study Hostel scored 100, indicating full physical function. Although this presented a seemingly accurate picture of the men's physical function, it did not express the nuances of some individuals' experience; that is, some men could undertake all the tasks listed in the Index, such as walking, grooming and so on, but they took 15 minutes to walk up the stairs, for example, or a long time to get to the toilet.

As stated above, it became apparent that the Barthel Index acted as an indicator of the hostels' ability to cater for disabled residents. The Comparison Hostel had better facilities than the Main Study Hostel (a lift and rooms on ground floor). This enabled residents with greater physical dysfunction (one in a wheelchair, one with multiple sclerosis, one with a fractured leg and one who was terminally ill) to live in the Comparison Hostel, and thus demonstrated many more men with a lower score, only 75% men scoring over 90. In the Main Study Hostel, where, to survive, an individual had to have higher physical function, 90% scored over 90. In summary, the higher the group scores of the Barthel Index, the *fewer* facilities for the disabled were available.

Hospital Anxiety and Depression Scale

Anxiety

The HAD Scale had been used in both hospital and community settings, but it had not previously been reported with homeless men. In discussion, some health professionals were doubtful about the use of the tool with this group. Some suspected that the men might give answers in order to gain attention, but this was disproved in the study. The scores of 46% of the Main Study Hostel sample fell within the normal range of scores, as did 65% of those in the Comparison Hostel. Twenty per cent were in the mid-range at the Main Study Hostel and 14% at the Comparison Hostel. Thirty-five per cent were in the high range at the Main Study Hostel and 20% at the Comparison Hostel.

The important feature about a high anxiety level is that, unlike a high depression level, it is susceptible to environmental factors. There is also a well-documented connection between anxiety and alcohol use. These factors were borne out in the study. Significant relationships were seen between high anxiety level and environmental factors such as length of residency, whether individuals wished to live in their hostel and individuals' feelings of well-being.

Depression

In the Main Study Hostel, only 38% of the sample had scores that fell within the normal range, 35% had scores within the middle range and 27% had scores lying within the high range. In contrast, the majority of the men in the Comparison Hostel – 71% – had scores that fell within the normal range, 18% within the mid-range and 11% in the high range. It is important to highlight that the express purpose of using the HAD depression tool was to isolate treatable clinical, biogenic depression by measuring 'anhedonia', the loss of the ability to experience pleasure. This condition has been found not to be susceptible to environmental factors or alcohol use. Comparison with these variables discovered that residents with a high depression score were found to be equally distributed throughout the impact of alcohol and length of stay comparisons.

These findings were presented to Dr R.P. Snaith at the University of Leeds, who developed the HAD tool. Dr Snaith estimated the occurrence of this form of non-reactive depression in the general population to be 5% or less. The levels in both hostels is, therefore, high, especially in the Main Study Hostel. This discovery became one of the most important findings of the study.

Impact of alcohol on lifestyle

The purpose of the Impact of Alcohol on Lifestyle Questionnaire was to measure the effects of alcohol consumption rather than the amount of consumption. This tool proved useful when the results were compared with other variables, particularly anxiety and prison record. Over half the men in the Main Study Hostel sample scored within the two higher score levels compared with just under half of the Comparison Hostel sample. These show a very high impact of alcohol on both populations. It is, however, important to point out that not all the men drank alcohol, or drank alcohol to excess.

Drug use

Several of the younger residents (aged under 25) used illegal substances, either by injection, orally or via smoking. Some of these men did not drink alcohol; some were even highly critical of alcohol abuse. Not everybody, however, was willing to discuss the issue.

Interventions

During the first 3 weeks of the study, almost all of those assessed required intervention. From the third to the seventh week of the field-work, the intervention rate became lower than the assessment rate. The first letter inviting residents to participate in the study was given out during the third week. A significant drop in assessment and intervention rates occurred between the sixth and eighth weeks, prompting the issuing of a second letter. This had a short-lived effect and was followed up by a final letter in the tenth week.

Interventions were divided in three categories, which are described in detail in Chapter 5. These were:

- treatments that were undertaken as an immediate measure when the man could not be referred to another agency;

- referrals;
- advocacy. Advocacy was defined as any action taken on behalf of a resident that supported his 'case' or helped him obtain aid that was not either a treatment or a referral.

Nine types of treatment were described, disinfestation and wound care being the most commonly employed. Eleven types of referral, mainly to GPs and the CPN, took place. Seventeen forms of advocacy were described, of which supporting telephone calls and arranging appointments were the most numerous.

Evaluation

Interviews with the health professionals

Twenty-three GPs received referrals from the project nurse; all were approached for interview, and 18 took part. The referrals were, in the main, felt to be appropriate and useful. The referrals had resulted in action and further referral, although only five had resulted in visits to the hostel by the doctor. None of the men with a high depression score were treated or referred for further intervention. Most of the doctors were sceptical about the benefits of starting treatment programmes with this client group, citing their unreliability as the main problem and the conditions of the hostels as the root of many of the physical and psychological problems.

Five district nurses received referrals from the project nurse (on six residents). All the nurses were interviewed. Three of the residents received specific nursing interventions, one being taken onto a district nurse's caseload for continuing monitoring. The two nurses who did not become involved stated that the GP did not think it appropriate for them to visit, one because the patient was thought to be violent, the second because the GP, who made regular visits to the hostels, was already seeing the patient.

Community nursing roles identified in the study

The study found that there were two main roles undertaken by district nurses. For the purpose of further study, it is suggested that these roles are relevant to all community nurses:

- *Proactive case-finder.* In this role (demonstrated by the project nurse), the community nurse acts as a 'generalist' able to make an initial assessment of individuals, followed by the relevant health treatment of immediate physical emergencies only, and/or referral to or advocacy with social and health agencies. The community nurse acting in this role can also undertake an ongoing monitoring of residents in an establishment.

- *Reactive specialist.* In this role, the community nurse performs particular specialist nursing tasks, such as ongoing wound or ulcer management, and the assessment and instigation of continuing or long-term care in response to referrals from mainly medical agencies.

Expert panel

The evidence gained from the responses and interventions made by the district nurses who received referrals from the project nurse was compared with the responses of an expert panel who were presented with five cases referred to district nurses and one that had not been referred. Whereas there was general agreement on what were appropriate interventions, all the expert panel's proposed actions in their responses were more wide ranging with regard to further intervention, support services and continued monitoring than were the responses of the district nurses who had actually received the referrals from the project nurse. Only two of the district nurses who received referrals from the project nurse actively included their patients in long-term monitoring.

Community psychiatric nursing team

Thirty-one residents were referred to the community psychiatric nursing team. Six of the men had left the hostel before being seen, and 25 were seen by the CPN. The team leader who was interviewed felt that the referrals had established a good working relationship between the project nurse and the team, and had improved the CPN team's access to residents. The team leader was doubtful, however, about the use of the HAD Scale and stated that the team focused mainly on psychotically ill residents.

Discussion

A discussion will now be presented that will highlight the lessons learned from the use of the particular methods chosen and also what are considered to be the most important findings.

The blend of methods

One of the defining features of this study was the combination of quantitative and qualitative elements. Quantitative evidence was collected, as were qualitative data from the project nurse's notes, which were arranged and coded into comments, themes and paradigms. The value of the use of both quantitative and qualitative approaches was that one set of data could support, or indeed challenge, the other. The discovery of two main groups of residents, for example, could be described in both the quantitative evidence and the paradigms. Similarly, the project nurse's qualitative observations regarding mental health morbidity were supported by statistically significant quantitative data.

The concentration of assessment and intervention

Patterns of recruitment

At the outset of the study, no strict timescale was set for the fieldwork. By counting the number of residents and allocating the number of interviews possible in a day, it was thought that the interviews would require 3 months, which proved to be the case. In a practice setting, however, the luxury of an open-ended timescale for interviewing and assessing patients is unlikely. As seen in Chapter 4, half of the interventions were in fact carried out in the first 3 weeks, and this was therefore a particularly important finding.

Visits to GPs and other health professionals

In Chapter 4, it was seen that a high proportion of the residents were attending their GPs on a regular basis, and in Chapter 5 a number of visits to the hostels by other health professionals were highlighted. These activities all focused on individuals with specific needs. In the case of the GPs, residents often visited them simply to collect a sickness certificate. These various health-related activities/visits could, if co-ordinated, provide an opportunity to the health professionals involved to monitor the health of these and possibly also other marginalized groups.

Use of referral as a monitoring tool

Although many of the project nurse's referrals were not followed through by residents, it was interesting to observe (see Chapter 6) how some of the GPs valued the referrals because they increased the clinical background information that could then be kept in the medical records. This demonstrates the intrinsic value of referrals, whether or not they are followed through by the potential patient.

Screening: possible limited use of observations and tests

Also described in Chapter 6 is how the GPs diagnosed three men as having hypertension. In Chapter 8, the discussion of the residents adaptive processes highlighted that aggressive screening (for example, taking blood or urine samples or monitoring other vital signs) for underlying morbidity was probably less effective than responding to what the patient wanted resolved. In this study, as a result of reading findings from research regarding homeless men, it was decided not to use a battery of observations and tests but to concentrate on eliciting the expressed need of the residents during the assessment. There may be a case, however, in future research and clinical projects with such groups of men for basic observations of blood pressure and urinalysis to be undertaken, in addition to eliciting expressed need through individual assessment.

Nursing roles

The proactive generalist

The project nurse, acting as a district nurse, demonstrated a wide variety of clinical and social skills and interactions. The importance of this general role was discussed in Chapter 5. The project nurse was able to identify both physical and psychiatric illness for ongoing referral, in comparison to the CPN's pattern of practice, which sought specific psychiatric illness. As a model for monitoring whole populations, in this and other groups, the project nurse's approach may be more effective as it is more wide ranging. Given the broad clinical experience of many community nurses and with an appropriate remit, future work should, however, concentrate on the physical and psychological competences required by nurses in conducting assessments rather than on their professional category.

The reactive specialist

Conversely, the district nurses who received referrals from the project nurse were seen (in Chapter 6) to act in a reactive specialist role, dealing, in the main, only with the specific presenting ailments. This contrasted with the responses of the members of the expert panel, described in Chapter 7, who suggested a more holistic repertoire of care involving the possible transfer of residents to other accommodation. The monitoring of a population of vulnerable or marginalized people might possibly be ineffective if district nurses acted only from referrals.

In a recent study of the effectiveness of the referral system as a means of identifying needs for district nursing, Worth et al (1995) state:

> There is little evidence of a proactive approach to the identification of need by district nurses at either individual or community level.

> Potential service users are discouraged from having direct access to
> district nursing advice and care, the GP acting as the primary
> gatekeeper. (p. xiii)

Worth et al's study later highlights the pressure to which district nurses
are subjected to by management, citing:

> unrealistic views of what district nurses can achieve, particularly in
> viewing a day's work in terms of numbers of visits, and workload in
> terms of the number of patients on the caseload. (p. 87)

When I visited the district nurses who received referrals at their health
centres, I found that they were extremely busy, with a great many
patients to see.

The combined burden of a busy caseload and management pressure
would seem to militate against a proactive, case-finding approach. It is
suggested therefore that co-ordinated hostel population monitoring,
were it to be instigated, would need to be planned strategically at a
management level rather than leaving it to individual nurses.

Since the study was completed two specialist community nurses for
the care of the homeless have been appointed in Glasgow. It is difficult
to know whether this study had a direct effect on this decision.
However, the study was funded by the Scottish Office Home and
Health Department (now the Scottish Executive), and I have been
fortunate enough to present not only the final report, but also several
presentations to various committees of experts and civil servants who
influence policy. The findings have also been disseminated to several
health service managers and community nurses.

Mental health: use of the HAD Scale

Throughout the study, psychiatric morbidity and psychological distress
featured highly. Among many of the men, the use of the HAD Scale
proved very relevant. In relation to seeking out residents with possible
biogenic depression, a large group of men were found, particularly in
the Main Study Hostel. The evidence of the expert witness who
devised the scale (see Chapter 7) suggested that many of these men
could be treated, and that their depression could have been a causative
factor in their homeless state rather than, as was the almost universal
professional assumption, that the men were depressed as a response to
their environment.

In the case of the anxiety scale, a strongly positive relationship was found between a high score on the HAD Scale and alcohol use problems. In addition, the group of mainly older men, who considered the hostels to be their home and preferred to have the companionship of other residents, tended to have a lower HAD anxiety score, whereas the group of mainly younger men, leading a more chaotic life, who did not feel at home, tended to score highly on the HAD anxiety scale. The HAD Scale thus assisted in the definition of these two groups.

It may be the case that if individuals suffering from depression in particular, as well as some of those suffering from anxiety, were treated systematically, a number of these people might be able to motivate themselves to take positive action. This might take the form of an increased exercise of personal responsibility and/or an uptake of mainstream services. It is difficult to see how an individual living in homeless accommodation and suffering from depression can move forward in his life without help.

Primary versus secondary care patterns of assessment

Further to the discussion on the specialist and generalist nursing roles of community nurses, the CPN's responses (see Chapter 6) demonstrated how the main focus of the psychiatric team's approach was to seek out residents suffering from psychotic illness, considering residents with other mental illness as being more able to seek help independently elsewhere.

This arrangement of priorities demonstrated a highly specialized, secondary (or hospital) care model of assessment as opposed to a primary care approach that would perhaps concentrate more on the effect that an individual's mental health was having on his ability to function normally. The primary care approach would, possibly, identify and be of more benefit to the individuals suffering from depression.

Theoretical and practical links

The care of the marginalized

The pattern of recruitment employed by the project nurse, a mixture of opportunistic encounters with the hostel residents and targeted letters, proved effective in reaching the sample population. It is suggested that this method, used alongside the assessment pack, which proved easy to administer, would be an effective way of monitoring other vulnerable and marginalized groups in society.

In Chapter 2, it was shown how the health and social profiles of the homeless, particularly their difficulties in accessing mainstream care, were also seen in other groups, for example prisoners, 'travelling people' and the single elderly. In Glasgow, there are several areas that have a concentration of elderly people, and many 'travelling people' in the city live on recognized sites. Using the same nursing assessment and intervention techniques that were used in this study may be of benefit to these individuals.

In a research study such as this one, it is important to specify a particular sample group, in the case of this study, single homeless men. It appears, however, from the study of the literature and the experience of the study, that the methods and approach would be relevant and appropriate for the study and care of other marginalized groups, including those mentioned above.

Residents' limited range of adaptation responses

In Chapter 8, an analysis of the residents' adaptive processes was presented using elements of Roy's (1980) theory of adaptation. The project nurse's experience, as witnessed in his fieldwork notes, indicated that many of the men had a limited capacity to adapt. This suggested that, when they encountered new problems, they did not make adaptations but responded using a limited range of responses. For example, many had problems associated with substance abuse, and they, with other residents, visited the project nurse on several occasions. These men were, however, unable to follow through any prescribed interventions or referrals made by the project nurse. In these cases, the project nurse witnessed residents engaging in a distressing circle of ineffectual activity.

It is suggested that one identifying factor of these and other vulnerable and marginalized people is their limited ability to adapt to situations with which other people may be able to cope. This limited capacity to respond was described in literature from the social anthropological field, where a recognition was made of individuals' limited 'loops' of response to social interaction rather than their possession of an infinite configuration of adaptations (Rapport 1993).

Sociological aspects – the groups

'Rootedness' versus 'uprootedness'

As described in Chapter 4 and discussed in Chapter 9, two broad groups of men were identified. The first, who tended to be younger, often led highly disorganized lives, often associated with substance abuse and admission to prison. These men did not, in the main, see the hostels as their home or their fellow residents as their preferred companions.

High anxiety scores were seen in this group. The second, older-age group tended to see the hostels as their home (having been residents for a longer time), to have lower anxiety levels and to prefer the company of their fellow residents to that of others such as their family.

Two points of interest emerged from the identification of these two groups. First, the sociological literature, particularly regarding deviancy theory, demonstrated patterns of antisocial behaviour with some single men (Sampson and Laub 1990). In the literature, there were conflicting views on whether these patterns resolved with age. In this study, it was not possible to assess whether the second, older group, was a different group in terms of the variables of admission to prison and family history, or the whether it represented the younger group grown old. Further sociological demographic study of these groups would be interesting.

Second, the literature discussed in Chapter 9 highlighted the concepts of the significance of place and individuals' 'rootedness' or 'uprootedness' (Godkin 1980). The two groups of men identified in this study could be classified as the 'rooted', older group and the 'uprooted', younger group.

There are practice implications for health professionals if they recognize and accept these two groups of residents. The emphasis on the rooted group of residents may be to assist them to achieve an improved and stable lifestyle where they are, and in strictly accurate terms they may not be considered 'homeless'. The second, uprooted, group may, however, require assistance in moving into more appropriate (for them) accommodation, as well as possible therapy for conditions such as alcoholism and depression.

Connected with the rooted group was a recognition in the study that some men wished to 'hand over' responsibility for their personal and health needs to other people. This 'passive' group may elicit conflicting responses from health professionals, who often try to empower patients to become more assertive and to make specific demands of the health services.

The study demonstrated practical methods of identifying the rooted and uprooted groups, including the HAD Scale (identifying anxiety and depression levels), the prison record and a record of the impact of alcohol use. Perhaps the simplest and best method was, however, asking the questions 'Where is home?' and 'How do you feel?' These questions produced a quick and accurate measure of the residents' health status and their perception of their residence.

Hopelessness – wrong assumptions?

The significance of the rooted and uprooted groups became apparent when considering the responses of the other group in this study, the health professionals. As described in Chapter 6, an almost universal pessimism was shown towards this group, even when nurses and doctors expressed positive support for them.

Health professionals' minimalist view

This pessimism resulted in a minimalist view of and response to hostel residents. Intervention tended to be very specific, concentrating on the presenting ailment. Given that one group (the uprooted) are often physically and psychologically frail (even though they tend to be the younger group) and may need assistance to move to more appropriate care and accommodation, and that the second (the rooted) group live in the hostels as their permanent home, this response seems inadequate by any standard.

In the Main Study Hostel, 12 widowers, mainly elderly, were discovered. When I was a district nurse in the same area as the Main Study Hostel, I had very few elderly men and widowers on my caseload. It is difficult not to conclude that the elderly men and widowers found in both hostels represent a significant proportion of that population in the local community. If this is the case, the question may be asked of whether the level of care provided to these elderly men, particularly those who have lost their wives, is comparable to, or indeed adequate compared with, that provided for the more numerous population of elderly widowed women.

Lack of influence of district nurses on the patients' environment

One of the main features of the district nurses' response was the lack of influence exerted on the residents' environment and a lack of any attempt by the nurses to seek alternative accommodation for the frail elderly. In contrast, Chapter 7 described the views of the expert panel when describing their possible response to referrals, which included the advocacy process to assist patients to obtain more suitable accommodation.

Taking into account the pressure of work that many individual health professionals are under, it would seem that the role of political and clinical advocacy, that is, influencing the standard of the residents' environment and the ongoing assessment of need and care of residents, particularly the frail, should also be a function of health boards and authorities.

By using multidisciplinary strategic planning, in conjunction with clinical assessment and monitoring, city-wide provision could be organized, with health centres acting in a pivotal role. This could be achieved by the extension of present primary care neighbourhood studies. Each health centre could identify the specific areas and buildings within its area where homeless and vulnerable groups of individuals resided.

Using small teams of community nurses, particularly district nurses and health visitors, with their broad-based assessment skills, and possibly using some of the methods described in this study, each group of residents and other individuals could be systematically assessed. These assessments could then form the basis of the establishment of specific care plans and could also possibly influence the purchasing of services and recruitment of staff.

Gender and professional class issues

There was evidence that health professionals treated hostels differently from other community settings. One district nurse (see Chapter 7) reported that 'her' GP did not like 'his' district nurses going into the hostels. Another thought that the elderly resident referred to her was violent, although the project nurse had not found or reported this. My experience as a male district nurse certainly mirrored this attitude. I have been asked, on occasions, to attend patients not on my caseload living on travellers' sites, because the female nurse did not want to go. No specific reason was given for these requests, but I assumed that it was for safety reasons.

There is no evidence that health professionals and others are more at risk in hostels, travellers' sites and other areas where marginalized people are gathered than they are elsewhere, yet there is caution, if not fear, surrounding professionals going into these areas. It would appear that some areas in the community are considered not fit for professionals, particularly female professionals in the female-dominated nursing profession, to enter. There is also evidence that part of the role of the GP as 'gate-keeper' (Worth et al 1995) is the protection and patronage of 'his' district nurses.

This discussion suggests not that these issues are universal but merely that they are present and/or may appear to influence decision-making and interaction with this group.

Individuals the study did not reach

It is important to highlight that, despite both opportunistic and targeted recruiting, a number of men did not seek assessment from or were not persuaded to take part by the project nurse. This demonstrated that, in spite of a systematic approach, it was not possible to reach everybody. Certainly, the hostel staff and the project nurse were aware that some men were too withdrawn to come forward, and others did not want contact for other reasons. In my experience with this and other marginalized groups, I have found that it sometimes takes many months to reach some individuals, gradually building up trust. Research studies are by their nature generally finite so future studies in this area should incorporate as much time as possible in order to achieve maximum coverage. From a practice perspective, the study's experience emphasizes the need to have a systematic community nursing assessment and monitoring of hostel residents so that relationships may be built up over time.

Having raised these issues, it should be stated that this study, by the use of systematic recruiting and the constant presence of the project nurse, did reach most of the Main Study Hostel population.

Preparing individuals for care

As stated above, the study did not reach some individuals, and, as reported in Chapter 5, the project nurse found that a large proportion of residents did not take up the appointments made for them. Chapter 6 included reflections on the GPs' comments, which also recognized that individuals from this group often did not follow through appointments. This non-compliance was not absolute: many men did respond to, for example, the tuberculosis screening as well as to the project nurse's referrals. Non-compliance, however, certainly does cause difficulties for professionals who are working with homeless men.

Attention is drawn to the other side of the issue, where the project nurse assisted residents to prepare for appointments both physically, for example, by giving them a bath, and psychologically, by interviewing residents and helping them to marshal their thoughts and needs into a more coherent form, both verbally and in writing. Many of the residents, prepared in this manner by the project nurse, did comply with appointments.

Assessment as intervention – a prerequisite for mainstream care

The preparation of residents by the project nurse for mainstream care puts the assessment process of these and other marginalized people into fresh perspective as the assessment actually becomes a form of intervention in itself. In Chapter 9 and the previous discussion, the suggestion was mooted that hostels could be 'no-go' areas for some professionals, or at least areas in which caution was shown regarding visits. By visiting the hostel and making assessments, the project nurse acted as a bridge for residents, helping to make them 'fit' for mainstream care.

If assessments are taken into account as performance measures, the five projects examined in Chapter 2 – particularly the London project described by Williams and Allen (1989) – in which concern was expressed about the success of the projects because of the difficulty in determining clinical outcomes, may now be viewed differently.

Recommendations for practice and future research

Recommendations for health service policy-makers

No claim can be made, of course, that an exact replication of this study – using the same validated tools, the same demographic questionnaire or the same nursing assessment – would serve a useful purpose. Each group of homeless people around the UK, for example, would present with a different age, ethnicity and social circumstance profile. Researchers in future studies would have to engage in exploratory work in their area to establish a more specific profile. For example, the sample in this study came mainly from the same ethnic/cultural group and even from the same area (Glasgow).

It can, however, be strongly recommended that the general method and approach, that is, the combination of a demographic profile with a nursing assessment and the use of validated tools containing score values, is generalizable. These score values can be combined with variables and values from the demographic profile to produce quantitative data. The quantitative data are enhanced by gathering qualitative data using incident diaries, case notes, the coding and grouping of themes and the use of paradigms. The combination of these methods produces, it is suggested, an extremely powerful description as it provides insight into the group while highlighting the experience of the individual.

The study demonstrated generalizable methods of community nursing practice, for this and other groups of marginalized clients, using assessment, referral and monitoring techniques and methods of recording both quantitative and qualitative data. Significant differences in practice patterns were demonstrated between district nursing using a case-finding approach, and nursing, which reacts to specific referral.

This current work has demonstrated practical ways of assessing the health needs of a group of homeless men – making an initial assessment of individuals, followed by the relevant treatment of any immediate physical emergencies, and/or referral to or advocacy on the part of social and health agencies. The community nurse is also capable of undertaking an ongoing monitoring role in an establishment where homeless men are housed.

Within a relatively few weeks, most of the pressing health needs of the men in the sample were discovered, half of the interventions taking place within the first 3 weeks. Using present resources and a management plan, all homeless accommodation could be targeted in this way.

The method of proactive assessment, intervention and monitoring used in this study could be applied in any institution of marginalized people in the community, for example in nursing homes and blocks of flats where there was a concentration of elderly and/or disabled. Each health centre could identify the hostels and other establishments housing vulnerable and marginalized people within its area. Programmes of assessment and monitoring could then be organized centrally.

Recommendations for health, social and housing service managers

As described in Chapter 2, there has, in recent years and especially since the National Health Service and Community Care Act 1990, been a policy drive to encourage joint working, particularly between health and social services but also with other public services such as housing (Department of Health 1994). Joint assessment, casework and funding lie at the centre of this development. It has, however, also been recognized that there is a considerable gap between rhetoric and practice (Lewis 1993).

Fundamental organizational problems exist that make it difficult for services to work together cohesively. Among the problems recognized are different strategic planning and bidding cycles, contradictory terms of reference, compulsory competitive tendering and the complications of each service having a purchaser/provider split (Goss 1996, Means 1996). Means (1996, p273), writing about housing and community care for older people, states:

> The danger of this situation is that it could undermine joint working at both central and local levels as different agencies jockey for position in the mixed economy debate while attempting to push costs into each other's budgets [known as shunting].

In terms of this study, it was found that although there was friendly co-operation between the individual workers in the different agencies (health, housing, social work and the voluntary sector), there was little evidence of strategic planning or management so that homeless men could gain access to an integrated package of health, housing and social care. In terms of the frail, elderly and widowed men, it can be suggested that such an approach would greatly assist these individuals, and it can thus be recommended that the increase of interprofessional strategic planning should take place at board/area and local authority level.

Patterns of practice

The study found that the community nurse can act in two distinct ways:

- as a case-finding generalist using a broad range of assessment methods and intervention skills; and/or
- as a reactive specialist with narrower responsibilities responding to mainly medical agencies.

The study has shown the importance and complementary nature of both of the above roles but recommends that the community nurse is allowed to perform each function.

Case-finding does not necessarily demand a long period of time when administered in a systematic fashion and therefore does not necessarily require costly extra resources.

Recommendations for service providers

The study found that many service providers held deep-seated preconceptions about homeless people, for example, that residents were not interested in their health. The study found, however, that many of the men were interested in their health, had treatable conditions, for example biogenic depression, and were prepared to attend appointments and undergo treatment.

The study also found that some service providers were prepared only to address the presenting complaint for each client without instituting ongoing monitoring. Most of the men were found to come into contact with primary health care teams on a regular basis, providing health services with an ideal opportunity to set up assessment and monitoring programmes.

It should be recognized that many individuals and groups will not take an assertive role in expressing their health and personal needs. Some people will prefer to hand over this responsibility to others while others are not capable of expressing themselves. Thus, whereas 'empowering' patients to express their specific needs as consumers, and therefore enabling nurses and others to react appropriately, may be a successful strategy in general, it may not be successful with particular individuals or groups.

It is recommended that those individuals who take a more passive role in terms of their health and personal needs may require a more proactive monitoring service that assists them to reach their full health potential.

Recommendations for future research

The following areas for further research can be identified:

- exploring the causes and effects of depression in homeless people, as well as the role of ill-health, as a causative factor, in people becoming homeless;
- evaluating projects that employ specialist community nurses and others using an integrated approach involving named district nurses along with a structured nursing assessment;
- examining the influences on assessment and intervention on outcome while following the progress of homeless and other marginalized people through their experience of the health services;
- investigating the number of elderly homeless men in a local and national demographic context and examining the practical choices they face in trying to maintain their health and lifestyle. A similar study of homeless people who are under 25 years of age is also recommended;
- replicating this study using the general approach and methods but with appropriate local adaptations to meet each group's needs:
  - with similar samples in other areas of Scotland and the UK;
  - with other marginalized groups such as travellers, single elderly people in their homes, ethnic minorities in deprived areas and refugees (in the UK);
  - with prisoners who have no fixed address.

Conclusion

The study described the residents of the Main Study Hostel, individually and collectively, through their eyes and within their own context. They were not only considered as a 'group' who were interacting, or not, with the health services; they were also examined as individuals within a group context. This, as far as it is known, is a unique approach. In district nursing, this has been the most systematic assessment and appraisal of needs and interventions for homeless men to date.

The study also systematically examined the use of short encounters, the nurse acting as a proactive case-finder and generalist, as a legitimate form of patient contact or technique for patient assessment with this group of homeless men. This pattern of practice was compared with the more normal practice of the nurse acting as a 'reactive specialist'.

The use of two theoretical frameworks provided a unique contribution. In particular, this is, as far as is known, the first time that a sociological perspective, including deviancy theory, has been used to highlight features of the interaction between this group and the health services. As a nurse, my professional tendency has always been to consider the individual. Using a sociological perspective has therefore been of great benefit, as the study has considered the men as a group, and has also studied some of the dynamics and rationale of group behaviour.

It is also the first time that Roy's (1980) adaptation theory has been used to analyse the actions and experience of homeless individuals. The theoretical analysis also provided insights into some of the problems that health professionals experienced in caring for this group, particularly with regard to identifying with the men and enacting an advocacy role.

The project was undertaken in a difficult but manageable community area. This will hopefully encourage further work in what are traditionally regarded as chaotic or marginalized settings. The study demonstrated the similarities between the study sample of homeless men and other groups of marginalized people, in addition to the implications for health professionals' practice of caring for these groups.

In particular, the study described the district nursing role of undertaking the physical and psychological assessment of the homeless men, witnessing and describing their experience and using this process to assist them physically and mentally to prepare for onward referral. When used in this manner, assessment may be seen as an intervention, that is, a vital prerequisite and preparation for access to mainstream care.

Perhaps the previous point encapsulates all the qualitative, quantitative and philosophical features of the study. It was found that the systematic measurement of the men's health needs and activities was useful. However, the presence of the project nurse, who spent time with the patients and bore witness to and described their experience, while assisting them to prepare for further care, was equally valuable.

In response to a survey by the Simon Community in London, a homeless person stated, with regard to health care professionals:

> They make you feel different. Don't respect you like a human being. Like a dog: it's wait, come, sit down.

> It's worse being homeless because society rejects you. They can't accept that you are ill. If you're homeless, you aren't taken seriously. (Leddington and Shiner 1991, p21)

It is hoped that this study has taken the homeless men seriously and shown methods of practice that can improve homeless people's experience of the health services, particularly nursing, within a context of care and respect.

It is also sincerely hoped that the story will not end here but that further research will build on the work described in this book. I would be delighted to assist any reader with further work and welcome any contact, so that the care provided to and experienced by homeless and other similarly marginalized people will become more effective in helping to address their health, social and personal needs.

Appendix I
Fieldwork pack

CONTENTS

Document one

Part One: Questionnaire and scores for statistical analysis

Part Two: Scores from validated and adapted assessment tools

Part Three: Nursing assessment

Document two

Part Four: Nursing intervention

Part Five: Evaluation of nursing intervention by researcher

DOCUMENT ONE

PART ONE: STATISTICAL QUESTIONNAIRE
PART TWO: VALIDATED ASSESSMENT TOOLS
PART THREE: NURSING ASSESSMENT

Resident's name   **Confidential**

Case ID no.   ☐☐

Date of first assessment   ☐☐☐☐☐☐

Date of first intervention   ☐☐☐☐☐☐

Intervention number   ☐☐☐

PART ONE: QUESTIONNAIRE AND SCORES FOR STATISTICAL
ANALYSIS IN MAIN STUDY HOSTEL AND COMPARISON HOSTEL.

Please ring around the appropriate response

For Office use only
COLUMNS 1–3
CASE ID

☐☐☐

COLUMNS 4–5
Project nurse approaches to resident (PA) limit of   4 ATTEMPTS

Resident approaches to project nurse (RA)

☐☐

PA RA

COLUMN 6
BLANK

1. Age (project nurse to take from records)   COLUMN 7–8

Under 18	01
18–25	02
26–40	03
41–50	04
51–60	05
61–70	06
71 and over	07

☐☐

AGE

2. Are you...?   COLUMN 9–10

Single	01
Married	02
Separated	03
Divorced	04
Widowed	05
Unable to answer	88
Doesn't want to answer	99

☐☐

MARITAL

COLUMN 11 BLANK
PART ONE
For Office use only
COLUMN 12–13

☐☐

3. How long have you been in this hostel?   STAYHOST

Under 3 months	01
3 months – 11 months	02
1–2 years	03
3–5 years	04

6–10 years   05
11 years and over   06
Don't know   77
Unable to answer   88
Doesn't want to answer   99

4. When was the last
    time you lived with your family?   COLUMN 14–15
    Under 3 months   01   □□
    3 months – 11 months   02
    1–2 years   03   FAMILY
    3–5 years   04
    6–10 years   05
    11 years and over   06
    Never lived with my family   07
    Don't know   77
    Unable to answer   88
    Doesn't want to answer   99

5. How long have you
    lived in homeless accommodation?   COLUMN 16–17
    Under 3 months   01   □□
    13 weeks – 5 months   02
    6 months – 11 months   03   HMLESTAY
    1–2 years   04
    3–5 years   05
    6–10 years   06
    11 years and over   07
    Don't know   77
    Unable to answer   88
    Doesn't want to answer   99   COLUMN 18 BLANK

6. When was the last time you worked?   COLUMN 19-20
    Currently working   01   □□
    Under 3 months   02
    3 months – 11 months   03   WORK
    1–5 years   04
    6–10 years   05
    11 years and over   06
    Never worked   07
    Don't know   77
    Unable to answer   88
    Doesn't want to answer   99

7. Are you registered
    with a GP?   COLUMN 21–22
          YES   01   ☐☐
          NO   02
    Don't know   77   GPREG
    Unable to answer   88
    Doesn't want to answer   99

If the response to Question 7 is 'NO', fill in
'Not applicable' to Questions 8, 9
and 10 and go to Question 11
If the response to Question 7 is 'YES', ask...

8. Is your GP?   COLUMN 23-24
    Within 1 mile   01   ☐☐
    2–3 miles   02
    Over 3 miles   03   GPDIST
    Not applicable   08
    Don't know   77
    Unable to answer   88
    Doesn't want to answer   99   COLUMN 25 BLANK

9. Are you currently receiving
    treatment from your GP?   COLUMN 26-27
          YES   01   ☐☐
          NO   02
    Not applicable   08   GPTREAT
    Don't know   77
    Unable to say answer   88
    Doesn't want to answer   99

If the response to Question 9 is 'NO', fill in
'Not applicable' to Question 10 and
go to Question 11
If the response to Question 9 is 'YES', ask...

10. Is the treatment from your GP for?   COLUMN 28–29
    Physical illness/condition   01   ☐☐
    Mental Illness   02
    Both   03   WATGPTRT
    Not applicable   08

Don't know   77
Unable to say answer   88
Doesn't want to answer   99

11. When was the last time you saw a GP?   COLUMN 30–31
    Within 3 months   01   □□
    3 months – 5 months   02
    6 months – 11 months   03   WHENGP
    1–2 years   04
    3–5 years   05
    Over 5 years   06
    Don't know   77
    Unable to answer   88
    Doesn't want to answer   99   COLUMN 32 BLANK

12. When was the last time you were a
    patient in hospital?   COLUMN 33–34
    In the last month   01   □□
    Under 3 months   02
    3 months – 11 months   03   WHENINPT
    1–2 years   04
    3–5 years   05
    Over 5 years   06
    Never been a patient in
        hospital?   07
    Don't know   77
    Unable to answer   88
    Doesn't want to answer   99

If the resident has 'Never been a patient in hospital',
fill in 'Not applicable' to Questions 13 and 14
and go to Question 15

13. How many admissions in the
    last 5 years for PHYSICAL ILLNESS?   COLUMN 35–36
        One   01   □□
        Two   02
        Three   03   ADMTPHYS
        Four   04
        Five   05
        Over Five   06
        Not applicable   08

Don't know	77
Unable to answer	88
Doesn't want to answer	99

COLUMN 37 BLANK

14. How many admissions in the
    last 5 years for MENTAL ILLNESS?   COLUMN 38–39

One	01
Two	02
Three	03
Four	04
Five	05
Over five	06
Not applicable	08
Don't know	77
Unable to answer	88
Doesn't want to answer	99

ADMTMENT

15. Do you currently attend a hospital
    outpatient clinic?   COLUMN 40–41

YES	01
NO	02
Don't know	77
Unable to answer	88
Doesn't want to answer	99

OPDATEND

If the response to Question 15 is 'NO', fill in
'Not applicable' to Question 16 and go to Question 17
If the response to Question 15 is 'YES', ask...

16. At the hospital outpatient clinic,
    do you receive treatment for a   COLUMN 42–43

Physical illness	01
Mental illness	02
Both	03
Not applicable	08
Don't know	77
Unable to answer	88
Doesn't want to answer	99

OPDTREAT

COLUMN 44 BLANK

17. Has a nurse visited you in this hostel? COLUMN 45–46

YES	01
NO	02
Don't know	77
Unable to answer	88
Doesn't want to answer	99

☐☐

NURHIST

18. Was the treatment from the nurse for? COLUMN 47–48

Physical illness/condition	01
Mental illness	02
Both	03
Not applicable	08
Don't know	77
Unable to say answer	88
Doesn't want to answer	99

☐☐

NURSTRT

If the response to Question 17 or 18 is 'NO'
or 'DON'T KNOW', fill in 'Not applicable'
to Questions 19 and 20 and go to Question 21
If the response to Question 17 is 'YES' ask...

19. Was the nurse a? COLUMN 49–50

District nurse	01
CPN	02
Health visitor	03
Other	04
Not applicable	08
Don't know	77
Unable to answer	88
Doesn't want to answer	99

☐☐

WATNURSE

COLUMN 51 BLANK

20. When did the nurse visit? COLUMN 52–53

Currently	01
Within 2 Years	02
Over 2 Years	03
Not applicable	08
Don't know	77
Unable to answer	88
Doesn't want to answer	99

☐☐

WHENURSE

21. In the last **two** years how many
    times have you visited Casualty ?

Never	01
Once	02
Twice	03
More than twice	04
Don't know	77
Unable to answer	88
Doesn't want to answer	99

COLUMN 54–55

□□

CASUALTY

22. Have you been in prison?

Never	01
Once	02
More than twice	03
Don't know	77
Unable to answer	88
Doesn't want to answer	99

COLUMN 56–57

□□

PRISON

COLUMN 58 BLANK

23. How do you feel health wise?

Well	01
Not very well	02
Ill	03
Very ill	04
Don't know	77
Unable to answer	88
Doesn't want to answer	99

COLUMN 59–60

□□

HOWUFEEL

24. Where would you like to live?

In a house or flat	01	Code	
In a hostel	02	Hospital	19
Other (please			
specify see code)	09	Sheltered housing	29
Don't know	77	Caravan	39
Unable to answer	88	No preference	49
Doesn't want			
to answer	99	Facetious reply	59

COLUMN 61–62

□□

LIKTOLIV

25. With whom would you like to live ?

Wife/family/partner	01
Friends	02
Other residents	03
With another group	04

COLUMN 63–64

□□

WHOULIV

By yourself   05
Don't know   77
Unable to answer   88
Doesn't want to answer 99

26. Where is 'home'?   COLUMN 65–66
    Here   01   ☐☐
    Where your family is   02
    Where you were born   03   WHEREHOM
    Somewhere else   04
    Nowhere   05
    Don't know   77
    Unable to answer   88
    Doesn't want to answer 99   COLUMN 67 BLANK

PART TWO: SCORES FROM VALIDATED AND ADAPTED
ASSESSMENT TOOLS

UNABLE to complete tools 888 or 88
DOES NOT WISH to complete tools 999 or 99

26. Barthel Index   COLUMN 68–70
    High score (nearer 100) = Good physical function ☐☐☐

    Low score (nearer 0) = Poor physical function   BARTIND

27. HAD Scale anxiety   COLUMN 71–72
    Normal range up to 7   ☐☐

                                                      HADANX

28. HAD Scale depression   COLUMN 73–74
    Normal range up to 7   ☐☐

                                                      HADDEP

29. Impact of alcohol

    Does not drink alcohol   777
    Some impact events on lifestyle   25–40

A number of impact events on lifestyle   40–60
(may be experiencing problems associated
   with alcohol use)
Considerable number of impact events on   60–120
lifestyle (may have a serious alcohol problem)

COLUMN 75–77

☐☐

ALCOHOL

30. Amount of smoking
How much do you smoke a day?
NONE   77
Pipe or 1–5 cigarettes or ¹/₄oz
   hand-rolling tobacco   05
6–10 cigarettes or 0.5 oz of hand-rolling tobacco 10
11–20 cigarettes or 1oz of hand-rolling tobacco   20
More than 20 cigarettes or more than 1oz of
   hand-rolling tobacco   30

COLUMN 78–79

☐☐

SMOKE

VALIDATED TOOLS OF ASSESSMENT

Functional assessment profile: The Barthel Index

Circle the score. Add the scores up. Place the total score in the box at the start of Part 2.

The Index should normally be applied through observation and, where necessary, from information from the resident or hostel staff

SELF-CARE INDEX	Can do without help	Can do with help	Can't do
1. Drinking from a cup	4	0	0
2. Eating	6	0	0
3. Dressing upper body	5	3	0
4. Dressing lower body	7	4	0
5. Putting on brace/ artificial limb	0	−2	0 (or N/A)
6. Grooming	5	0	0
7. Washing/bathing	6	0	0
SPHINCTER CONTROL			
8. Controlling urination	10	5	0 incontinent
9. Controlling bowels	10	5	0 incontinent
MOBILITY INDEX			
10. Getting in and out of chair	15	7	0
11. Getting on/off toilet	6	3	0
12. Getting in/out of bath/shower	1	0	0
13. Walking 25 yards on the level	15	10	0
14. Walking up/down one flight	10	5	0
15. Propelling/pushing wheelchair	5	0	0 (or N/A)

SCORE ☐☐☐

Reference: Mahoney and Barthel (1965)

Hospital Anxiety and Depression (HAD) Scale

Scale is scored in two parts: ANXIETY(A) and DEPRESSION (D)
Add the individual scores. Place the TWO total scores in the boxes at
the start of part 2.
If the resident is UNABLE to answer, place 88 in the score box
If the resident DOES NOT WISH to answer, place 99 in the score box

(i) I feel tense or wound up: A3

Most of the time	3
A lot of·the time	2
From time to time, occasionally	1
Not at all	0

A ☐

(ii) I feel as if I am slowed down: D3

Nearly all the time	3
Very often	2
Sometimes	1
Not at all	0

D ☐

(iii) I still enjoy the things I used
to enjoy: D0

Definitely as much	0
Not quite so much	1
Only a little	2
Hardly at all	3

D ☐

(iv) I get a frightened feeling like
butterflies in the stomach: A0

Not at all	0
Occasionally	1
Quite often	2
Very often	3

A ☐

(v) I get a frightened feeling as if
      something awful is about to happen: A3

    Very definitely and quite badly   3
    (Yes, but) not too badly   2
    A little, but it doesn't worry me   1
    Not at all   0

             A ☐

(vi) I have lost interest in my appearance: D3
    Definitely   .   3
    I don't take so much care as
      I should   2
    I may not take quite as
      much care (as I did)   1
    I take just as much care as ever   0

             D ☐

(vii) I can laugh and see the funny side of
    things: D0
    As much as I always could   0
    Not quite so much now   1
    Definitely not so much now   2
    Not at all   3

             D ☐

(viii) I feel restless as if I have to be
on the move: A3

Very much indeed   3
Quite a lot   2
Not very much   1
Not at all   0

             A ☐

(ix) Worrying thoughts go through
    my mind: A3
      A great deal of the time   3
      A lot of the time   2
      From time to time but not too often   1
      Only occasionally   0

                A ☐

(x) I look forward with enjoyment
    to things: D0:
      As much as I ever did   0
      Rather less than I used to   1
      Definitely less than I used to 2
      Hardly at all   3

                D ☐

(xi) I feel cheerful: D3
      Not at all   3
      Not often   2
      Sometimes   1
      Most of the time   0

                D ☐

(xii) I get sudden feelings of panic: A3:
      Very often indeed   3
      Quite often   2
      Not very often   1
      Not at all   0

           A ☐

(xiii) I can sit at ease and feel relaxed: A0:

    definitely   0
    usually   1
    not often   2
    not at all   3
      A

(xiv) I can enjoy a good book, radio or TV programme: D0:

often	0
sometimes	1
not often	2
very seldom	3
D	

ANXIETY SCORE   DEPRESSION SCORE

Reference: Zigmond and Snaith (1983)

ADAPTED TOOL OF ASSESSMENT

Impact of Alchohol Use on Lifestyle Questionnaire

Adapted from the work of Dr Harvey Skinner (1982), Addiction Research
Foundation, Toronto, Canada (Drug and Alcohol Use Questionnaires)

Ring around the scores. Place the total score in the box at the start of part 2.
If you are UNABLE to complete the questionnaire, place 888 in the score box.
If the resident DOES NOT WISH to complete the questionnaire, place 999 in
the score box.

1. Do you drink alcohol?   YES   (010)   ☐ ☐ ☐
                                       NO   (777)

    If NO, stop questionnaire
    If YES, please proceed with questionnaire

2. How many days a week   1 2 3 4 days (05)   ☐ ☐
    do you usually drink alcohol?   5 6 7 days   (15)

3. Do you always drink alcohol   Yes   (05)   ☐ ☐
    when you get your money?   Not always   (00)

4. How much alcohol do you
    drink in one day (in units)?   1-5 units   (05)   ☐ ☐
    (A unit is half a pint of beer   6-10 units   (10)
    or a dram of spirit)   11+ units   (20)

5. How much do you spend on drinking alcohol a week? (Question asked to
    test the accuracy of answer 4, no score required)

6. Have you ever been hospitalized   YES   (10)   ☐ ☐
    or been to the doctor because of NO   (00)
    drinking alcohol?

7. Has drinking alcohol ever caused
    you to be injured?   YES   (10)   ☐ ☐
                                      NO   (00)

8. Have you ever engaged in illegal
    activities to get alcohol?   YES   (10)   ☐ ☐
                                      NO   (00)

9. Have you ever been arrested
    following drinking alcohol?   YES   (10)   ☐☐
                                    NO   (00)

10. Do you drink more alcohol
    or less since living here?   Less   (00)   ☐☐
                                    Same   (05)
                                    More   (10)

11. Do you think your drinking
    alcohol has affected your life? A Lot   (10)   ☐☐
                                    A Little   (05)
                                    Not at all (00)

12. Does your drinking alcohol affect
    your relationships with others   A Lot   (10)   ☐☐
                                    A Little   (05)
                                    Not at all (00)

                                    SCORE   ☐☐☐

Smoking use questionnaire

Ring around the scores. Place the total score in the box at the start of part 2.
If you are UNABLE to complete the questionnaire place 88 in the score box.
If the resident DOES NOT WISH to complete the questionnaire place 99 in the
score box.

1. Do You Smoke ?   YES   (00)   ☐☐
                                    NO   (77)

    If NO, stop questionnaire
    If YES, please proceed with questionnaire

2. How much do you smoke a day?
    Pipe or 1–5 cigarettes or ¼ oz hand-rolling tobacco (05)   ☐☐
    6–10 cigarettes or 0.5 oz of hand-rolling tobacco   (10)
    11–20 cigarettes or 1 oz of hand-rolling tobacco   (20)
    More than 20 cigarettes or more than 1 oz of
        hand-rolling tobacco   (30)

3. How much do you spend on smoking a week?
    (Question asked to test the accuracy of the last question; no score required)

                                    TOTAL   ☐☐

PART THREE: NURSING ASSESSMENT

Brief objective measures for the determination of mental status in the aged

This questionnaire is ONLY FOR RESIDENTS OF 60 YEARS AND OVER.
It is used as a GUIDE ONLY and may assist when referring the resident to
medical services. Other factors may prevent the resident answering correctly,
e.g. social isolation or questions' lack of relevance.

Allocate ONE mark for each correct answer.

1. What is the name of this place?

2. Where is it located (address)?

3. What is today's date?

4. What is the month now?

5. What is the year?

6. How old are you?

7. When were you born (month)?

8. When were you born (year)?

9. Who is the Prime Minister ?
   (Modified from the USA, 'the President')

10. Who was the Prime Minister before him?
    (Modified from the USA, 'the President')

MARK OUT OF 10
☐☐

Reference: Khan et al. (1960)

Notes for the project nurse on the semi-structured interview

- Please try to create as relaxed and private an atmosphere as possible for the resident
- Do not rush the resident
- The headings and questions are to help you focus your conversation with the resident onto key nursing assessment areas
- Try to guide the conversation with your questions in the order given on this form. It is, however, accepted that the resident may return to subjects or decide to talk about subjects in his own way and in his own time.
- Do not write at length on this form
- Under each question write your comments in short but easily readable sentences or phrases.
- Try to use one line per comment
- Number each separate comment

Example: Eliminating
Check with the hostel staff for evidence of incontinence
1. Hostel staff give him a change of sheets 2–3 times a week

Do you have any problems passing water? Any other urinary problems?
1. Takes him 10 minutes to micturate
2. Dribbles afterwards

Do you have any problems opening your bowels?
Any other anal or rectal problems?
1. No bowel motion for five days. This happens often
2. Painful when passing stools, sometimes bleeds

Incident Diary (comments, themes and paradigms)

If the resident tells you something you would like to record in more detail, please record this in the incident diary.
Please make sure to cross-reference properly. The paradigm should be accompanied by the assessment date, the resident's name, the case ID No and the intervention number.

Themes. As you interview the residents, you may come across recurring themes of a clinical and/or social nature
Please record these in the comments, themes and paradigms book and cross-reference as above.

NURSING ASSESSMENT
SEMI-STRUCTURED INTERVIEW

The project nurse is a qualified district nurse and is expected to use his clinical judgement to augment the semi-structured interview. The questions on this page may need to be supported by evidence from the hostel staff and others who know the resident.

Maintaining a safe environment
Risk factors
Prompt: Does he have accidents in his room? Does he fall?

Getting lost
Prompt: Do the staff find the resident wandering, sometimes getting lost? Do the staff ever have to supervise him?

Communication and speech
Prompt: Is the resident understood? With difficulty ?
Prompt: Does he convey his wishes and needs?

Hearing and understanding
Prompt: Does the resident have a hearing aid? Does he have a problem hearing the project nurse?
Prompt: Does he usually understand oral communication?
Prompt: Does he have a limited understanding of oral communication?

The questions in the semi-structured interview are also there to discover the resident's health, social experience and aspirations, and the barriers that may affect his health and access to services. Some of the questions are accompanied by directions. This sometimes includes consulting with hostel staff and other professionals who may know him. This should be carried out after the interview.

Breathing
Prompt: Can you sleep lying flat?
Prompt: Do you have any other difficulties with breathing?

Eating and drinking
N.B. Does the resident fit his clothes? Does he have dentures?
Prompt: How many meals a day do you eat?
Prompt: How much fluid intake a day?
Prompt: Do you have difficulties eating and drinking?

Eliminating
Check with hostel staff for evidence of incontinence
Prompt: Do you have any problems passing water? Any other urinary problems?
Prompt: Do you have any problems opening your bowels? Any other anal or rectal problems?

Personal cleansing/dressing
Is the resident infested? Check with hostel staff as well as examining the resident
Prompt: Do you have a change of clothes?
Prompt: Do you have difficulty keeping clean?

Controlling body temperature
Is the resident appropriately dressed?
Prompt: Do you have trouble keeping warm?

Mobilizing
Check with the resident's Barthel assessment
Does the resident use a Zimmer frame or other aid?
Does the resident have any other mobilizing problems? Check with hostel staff
Prompt: Do you have leg ulcers? Check the resident's legs
Prompt: Do you have any foot problems?
Prompt: Do you have any other mobilizing difficulties?

Working and recreation
From the statistical questionnaire, you will know whether the resident works
If he does work, it may be relevant to ask details of his employment but ONLY if the resident wishes.
Ask about the resident's recreational activities

Sleeping
Prompt: Do you have any problems sleeping?
Prompt: Do you have anything else you want to tell me about?

Record any other relevant physical factors

Record any other psychological factors, such as the resident's mental state during the interview

Record any other socio-cultural, environmental or politico-economic factors, such as a recent bereavement, recent discharge from prison or long-term care, recent loss of income, recently becoming homeless or recent discharge from hospital

Reference: Roper et al (1990)

Finally, in this part, ask the resident the following questions. They will help to focus what the questionnaire and assessment have discovered and combine this with what the resident thinks and wants

What problems do you have at present?

1.

2.

3.

What would you like done for you?

1.

2.

3.

Does this resident need nursing and/or medical intervention?

If the answer is NO, the interview may stop here
If the answer is YES, go on to PART FOUR

DOCUMENT TWO

PART FOUR: INTERVENTION
PART FIVE: EVALUATION

Resident's name   Confidential

Case ID no.   ☐☐

Date of first assessment   ☐☐☐☐☐☐

Date of first intervention   ☐☐☐☐☐☐

Intervention number   ☐☐☐

PART FOUR: NURSING INTERVENTION

Planning for intervention by project nurse
Roy's (1980) adaptation model

This part of the study examines the resident's needs and problems as areas where adaptions may be made, the purpose being to help the project nurse to focus, reflect and form a professional judgement

In this part of the study, you will be considering the information gained in the assessment, with a view to nursing intervention

At this stage you will be presented with TWO options:

A. Having decided that the resident will need intervention, it may be appropriate to finish the assessment interview at this stage, returning to him after you have reflected and/or engaged in professional liaison, gained advice and developed a proposed plan of intervention for the resident's approval. If this is the case thank the resident and tell him that you will come and see him later.

B. Having decided that the resident will need intervention, it may be appropriate for the resident to remain with you while you plan the nursing intervention with him. If this is the case, tell the resident that this is your intention and seek his co-operation.

The project nurse will form his professional judgement from four areas.

1. The formal assessment
2. The chance or short encounter
3. Observation
4. Information from others who know the resident, particularly the hostel staff

This is a framework to guide the project nurse in his professional reflection and judgement. As you get to know the resident, you may develop his profile by using this reflective tool.

References: Aggleton and Chalmers (1986); Roy (1980)

1st STAGE: Does the resident's health experience or behaviour in any of the four adaptive modes give cause for concern?

A. *Physiological adaptive mode*
Consider whether the resident suffers from physical problems that need intervention or adaptation from the health services. Examples may be sleeplessness, confusion, social withdrawal, malnutrition, vomiting, constipation, incontinence, dehydration, oedema and hypothermia

B. *Self-concept adaptive mode*
Consider whether the resident experiences self-concept (internal) barriers that affect his ability to access health care and services. Is he experiencing a sense of physical loss or anxiety? Does he feel powerless or socially disengaged? Does this make him feel that he cannot do anything about his health?

C. *Role function adaptive mode*
Consider whether the resident feels a failure because he feels that he has failed as a father, husband, family member or working member of society. You may not get this information by direct questioning: he may tell you about this area while speaking about his family or life before he came to the hostel

D. *Interdependency adaptive mode*
Consider whether the resident feels rejected by others. Does he feel alienated from others, particularly his family and dependants? Does he feel lonely?
N.B. Does he have experiences and feelings of rejection in relation to the health services?

Having examined these four areas, is there any need deficit that could benefit from the intervention and/or adaptation of health services?

2nd STAGE: Are the resident's adaptation problems due to?

i. Focal stimuli
This refers to factors or external barriers regarding human elements such as present services, facilities and personnel encountered, for example hostel facilities, his fellow residents and the present services he may be receiving.

ii. Contextual stimuli
This refers to factors or external barriers regarding the physical environment in which he lives, for example the living space, ambient temperature and distance to the toilet.

iii. Residual stimuli
This refers to factors or internal barriers emanating from the resident, his beliefs and attitudes to health services.
Does he feel that he has received prejudicial treatment from the health services?
Does he feel unable to avail himself of the health services?
What are his expectations of the health services to help him?

Referring to 'Where would you like to live?' and 'Where is Home?' above, do the answers affect the resident's expectations of his lifestyle and health services?

Mark interventions as follows...
    (T) TREATMENT
    (R) REFERRAL
    (A) ADVOCACY

- Use ONE LINE for each intervention
- NUMBER each intervention

Most interventions will involve 'altering stimuli', for example changing or initiating a service. Some interventions will demonstrate 'extending the resident's adaptation', for example a resident attending an appointment you have made for him (RA).

Express the interventions as follows:

Examples:
1. Incident diary re recent bereavement   (D)
2. Dressed suppurating left leg ulcer   (T)
3. Letter to GP re left leg ulcer   (R)
4. Letter to DN re left leg ulcer   (R)
5. Supporting letter of introduction to outpatient sister   (A)
6. Resident attended outpatient appointment arranged
    by the project nurse   (A)(RA)

Fill in blank sheets as follows:

DATE:
TIME:
SESSION:
PROBLEM: INTERVENTIONS:

DATE:
TIME:
SESSION:
PROBLEM :   INTERVENTIONS:

PART FIVE: EVALUATION OF NURSING INTERVENTION BY RESEARCHER

Semi-structured interviews of health professionals

Health professional 1

Case ID of health professional

☐☐☐

District nurses' numbers start with 1
GPs' numbers start with 2
Community psychiatric nurses' numbers start with 3

NAME:

PROFESSION:

ADDRESS:

What did you do as a result of the nursing referral you received regarding this resident?

How did you come to make these decisions?

Did you have any difficulty putting your plan into action?

How easy was it to find your patient?

What was your opinion of his physical and mental status?

Was the referral appropriate?

Did you find any other reasons why this patient needed your specialist attention?

If so, what were these?

Have you looked after homeless residents before?

Have you any views regarding delivery of an effective service to them?

Any other comments?

Health professional 2

Case ID of health professional

☐☐☐

District nurses' numbers start with 1
GPs' numbers start with 2
Community psychiatric nurses' numbers start with 3

NAME:

PROFESSION:

ADDRESS:

What did you do as a result of the nursing referral you received regarding this resident?

How did you come to make these decisions?

Did you have any difficulty putting your plan into action?

How easy was it to find your patient?

What was your opinion of his physical and mental status?

Was the referral appropriate?

Did you find any other reasons why this patient needed your specialist attention?

If so, what were these?

Have you looked after homeless residents before?

Have you any views regarding delivery of an effective service to them?

Any other comments?

Appendix II:
Sample letters

Letter to residents
Date:

Dear Mr [Hostel resident],

As you may be aware, I have been meeting with residents recently to talk about their health and other matters that concern them. So far, I have met about 50 residents and have been able to help or advise over 30.

During the next few days, I would like to meet with you and other residents living on the first floor to have a chat. Those living on other floors will receive a similar letter in a few weeks.

I hope that our meeting will not only help you, but will also help to improve services to this hostel.

I will be here most mornings in the medical room on the ground floor and would be happy to meet you at any time, either in the medical room or in your own room. If you cannot find me please ask the hostel staff.

Thank you for your time. I look forward to meeting you.

Yours sincerely

John S. Dreghorn
District Nurse

Letter to GPs and nurses
Case ID No.:
Intervention No.:
Date:

Dear [GP or nurse]

I saw   who is a resident at this establishment.

I would like to refer this man to you following an assessment by myself on

I would like to bring the following details to your attention:

I hope you find these details useful. If you wish to write to me, please do so at the above address. If you wish to telephone me, you may use either of the above telephone numbers.

Thank you for your consideration in this matter.

Yours sincerely

John Dreghorn RGN DipPS DipDN
District Nurse working with Greater Glasgow Health Board
Community Primary Health Care Unit, Community Nursing and
Glasgow Caledonian University, Department of Nursing and
Community Health.

References

Abrams P, Brown R (Eds) (1984) UK Society: Work, Urbanism and Inequality. London: Weidenfield and Nicholson.

Acheson D, for the London Health Planning Consortium. (1981) Primary Health Care in Inner London. London: HMSO.

Aggleton P, Chalmers H (1986) Nursing Models and the Nursing Process. London: Macmillan.

Akinsanya JA (1987) The life sciences in nursing: development of a theoretical model. Journal of Advanced Nursing 12(3): 267–74.

Ambrosio E (1991) Poor housing, poor health. Canadian Nurse 87(5): 22–4.

Anderson G (1984) Changing attitudes, taking risks. Nursing Times 80(2): 19–20.

Andrews FM, Withey SB (1976) Social Indicators of Wellbeing. New York.

Antrobus M (1987) The neglected sex. Nursing Times 83(6): 31–3.

Aronson E (1991) The Social Animal. 6th edn. New York: WH Freeman.

Association of Community Health Councils (1989) Homelessness: The Effects on Health. London: CHC.

Atkinson J (1987) I just exist. Community Outlook (Nov): 12–15.

Atkinson J (1989) A flexible friend. Community Outlook (Jun): 4–6.

Atkinson J (1997) A Descriptive and Evaluative Study of District Nursing Intervention with Single Homeless Men from a Private Hostel in Glasgow. PhD thesis, Glasgow Caledonian University.

Atkinson J, Thompson R (1989) Homelessness and health. Nursing Standard 3(43): 51.

Badger F, Cameron E, Evers H (1988a) Caseloads under review. Health Service Journal 98: 1327–1329.

Badger F, Cameron E, Evers H (1988b) Nursing in perspective. Health Service Journal 98: 1362–3.

Baine S, Benington J (1992) Changing Europe: Challenges Facing the Voluntary and Community Sectors in the 1990's. London: National Council for Voluntary Organisations Community Development Foundation.

Baly ME (Ed) (1981) A New Approach to District Nursing. London: William Heinemann.

Baly ME (1987) The History of the Queen's Nursing Institute. London: Croom Helm.

Barker P (1989) Reflections on the philosophy of caring in mental health. International Journal of Nursing Studies 26(2): 131–41.

Barnes C (1991) Disabled People in Britain and Discrimination: A Case for Anti-discrimination Legislation. London: Hurst.

Barry A, Carr Hill R, Glanville J (1991) Homelessness and Health: What Do we Know? What Should Be Done? Discussion Paper No. 84. York: University of York Centre for Health Economics.

Bayliss E, Logan P (1987) Primary Health Care for Homeless Single People in London: A Strategic Approach. Report of the Health Sub Group of the Joint Working Party on Single Homelessness in London. London: Single Homeless in London/London Borough of Hammersmith and Fulham.

Beauchamp T, Perlin S (1978) Ethical Issues in Death and Dying. Englewood Cliffs, NJ: Prentice Hall.

Benner P (1984) From Novice to Expert: Excellence and Power in Clinical Nursing Practice. Menlo Park, CA: Addison-Wesley.

Berkman B (1978) Mental health and ageing – a review of the literature for clinical social workers. Clinical Social Work Journal 6: 230–45.

Berthoud R, Casey B (1988) The Cost of Care in Hostels. London: Policy Studies Institute/DHSS.

Bishop AH, Scudder JR (1990) The Practical, Moral, and Personal Sense of Nursing. New York: State University of New York Press.

Black ME, Scheuer MA, Victor C, Benzeval M, Gill M, Judge K (1991) Utilisation by homeless people of acute hospital services in London. British Medical Journal 303(6808): 958–61.

Black Housing (1989) Black People and Housing. Black Housing 5(11): 5-8.

Bonnerjea L, Lawton J (1987) Homeless in Brent. London: Policy Studies Institute.

Bordieu P (1990) The Logic of Practice. Cambridge: Polity Press.

Boss M (1979) Existential Foundations of Medicine and Psychology. New Jersey: Jason Aronson.

Bowers J (1988) Review essay on discourse and social psychology: Beyond attitude by Jonathon Pott and Margaret Wetherell. British Journal of Social Psychology 27: 185–92.

Brickner PW (1986) Homeless persons and health care. Annals of Internal Medicine 104(3): 405–9.

Brimacombe M (1987) Who's Homeless Now? Shelter 21st Anniversary Publication. London: Shelter.

Brimacombe M (1990) Prison: 'home' for the mentally ill. Housing 26(1): 10–13.

British Broadcasting Corporation (BBC2) (1987) A Nice Way to Treat People: An Open Space Film about Health Care and Homelessness. Transcript of programme, 12 August.

Buck MH (1991) 'The physical self' and 'The personal self'. In Roy C, Andrews HA (Eds) The Roy Adaptation Model – the Definitive Statement. Norwalk, CT: Appleton and Lange, pp 281–310, 310–35.

Burnard P (1990) Counselling Skills for Health Professionals. London: Chapman and Hall.

Burnard P (1991) A method of analysing interview transcripts in qualitative research. Nurse Education Today 1(11): 461–6.

Buttimer A, Seamon D (Eds) (1980) The Human Experience of Time and Space. London: Croom Helm.

Caffey J (1946) Multiple fractures in the long bones of infants suffering from chronic subdural haematoma. American Journal of Roentgenology 56(2): 173–6.

Calderwood R (1989) Strathclyde Social Trends. 2nd Edn. Glasgow: Strathclyde Regional Council.

Calsyn RJ, Morse GA (1991) Predicting chronic homelessness. Urban Affairs Quarterly 27(1): 155–64.

Carper BA (1978) Fundamental patterns of knowing in nursing. Advances in Nursing Science 1(1): 13–23.

Checkland O, Lamb M (Eds) 1982 Health Care as Social History: The Glasgow Case. Aberdeen University Press.

CIBA Foundation (1973) Medical Care of Prisoners and Detainees. London: Associated Scientific Publishers.

Clapham D (1991) In Smith SJ, McGuckin A, Knill Jones R (Eds) Housing for Health. Harlow: Longman.

Connelly J, Roderick P, Victor C (1991) Is housing a public health issue? A survey of Directors of Public Health. British Medical Journal 302(6769): 157–60.

Conrad P, Schneider JW (1980) Deviance and Medicalization: From Badness to Sickness. St Louis, MO: CV Mosby.

Courtney R (1988) Bleak future for the homeless. Scope (112): 6–8.

Crane M (1990) Old, homeless and unwanted. Nursing Times 86(21): 44–6.

Crisis (1992) Annual Report of the 'Crisis' Charity. London: Crisis.

Daly G (1989) Homelessness and health: views and responses in Canada, the United Kingdom and the United States. Health Promotion 4(2): 115–28.

Dant T, Deacon A (1989) Hostels to Homes? The Rehousing of Single Homeless Men. Aldershot: Avebury.

Davis DS (1986) Nursing: an ethic of caring. Humane Medicine 2(1): 19–25.

Defoe D (1753) A Tour thro' the Whole Isle of Great Britain. 5th edn. Printed for S Birt and others. London.

Department of the Environment (1987) Homeless Statistics for England 1st Half 1987. London: DoE.

Department of Health (1994) Implementing Caring for People: Community Care Packages for Older People. London: DoH.

Department of Health and Social Security (1985) Service Planning for the Single Homeless. HC(FP)(5)10. London: HMSO.

Diener E (1984) Subjective wellbeing. Psychological Wellbeing 95(3): 542–75.

Donaghue H (1989) The Great Eastern Hotel Project. Branch Report. Glasgow: British Red Cross.

Douglas RNC (1987) The house and lineage of David – history of a practice. Glasgow Medical Journal (Jun).

Downes D, Rock P (1982) Understanding Deviance. Oxford: Clarendon Press.

Downie R, Telfer E (1980) Caring and Curing. London: Methuen.

Drake M, O'Brien M, Biebuyck T for the Department of the Environment (1981) Single and Homeless. London: HMSO.

Drake M, Littler T, Canter D (1989) The Faces of Homelessness in London: Interim Report to the Salvation Army. Surrey: University of Surrey, Department of Psychology/Salvation Army.

Drennan V, Stearn J (1986) Health visitors and homeless families. Health Visitor 59(11): 340–2.

Dunn WR, Hamilton DD (1986) The critical incident technique – a brief guide. Medical Teacher 8(3): 207–15.

Edwards K (1986) Passing the buck. New Society 76(1216): ii.

El Kabir J, Nyiri P, Ramsden SS, Bridgewater J (1989) A mobile surgery for single homeless people in London. British Medical Journal 298(6670): 372–4.

Fawcett J (1992) Conceptual models and nursing practice: the reciprocal relationship. Journal of Advanced Nursing 17: 224–8.

Featherstone P, Ashmore C (1988) Health surveillance project among single homeless men in Bristol. Journal of the Royal College of General Practitioners 38(313): 353–5.

Flanagan JC (1954) The critical incident technique. Psychological Bulletin 51(4): 327–58.

Flynn BC (1988) An action research framework for primary health care. Nursing Outlook (Nov/Dec): 316–18.

Foucault M (1973) The Birth of the Clinic: An Archaeology of Medical Perception. London: Tavistock Publications.

Garside PL, Grimshaw RW, Ward FJ for the Department of the Environment (1990) No Place Like Home: The Hostels Experience. London: HMSO.

George L (1981) Subjective wellbeing: conceptual and methodological issues. Annual Review of Gerontology and Geriatrics 2: 345–82.

Glasgow Caledonian University (1992) Course notes for District Nursing students.

Glasgow Council for Single Homeless (1984) Annual Report. Glasgow: GCSH.

Glasgow Council for Single Homeless (1989a) The Glasgow Stopover. Glasgow: GCSH.

Glasgow Council for Single Homeless (1989b) Turning Points – a Strategy on Single Homelessness in Glasgow. Glasgow: GCSH.

Glasgow Council for Single Homeless (1989c) Annual Report. Glasgow: GCSH.

Glasgow Council for Single Homeless (1990a) Single Homeless and Housing Need in Glasgow – a Report on a GCSH Survey of Hostel Residents. Glasgow: GCSH.

Glasgow Council for Single Homeless (1990b) Annual Report. Glasgow: GCSH.

Glasgow Council for Single Homeless (1991) Developments in Single Homelessness Annual Report. Glasgow: GCSH.

Glasgow District Council and Shelter Scotland (1991) Homeless Policy, Procedures and Practice. Glasgow: GDC.

Godkin MA (1980) Identity and place: clinical applications based on notions of rootedness and uprootedness. In Buttermer A, Seamon D (Eds) The Human Experience of Space and Place. London: Croom Helm, p 73.

Goffman E (1961) Stigma Notes on the Management of a Spoiled Identity. London: Penguin.

Goldberg D (1985) Identifying psychiatric illness among general medical patients. British Medical Journal 291(6489): 161–2.

Gosling J (1989) One Day I'll Have My Own Place To Stay ... Young Homeless People Write about their Lives. London: Central London Social Security Advisers Forum/Shelter.

Gosling J (1990) Young Homeless: A National Scandal. London: Young Homeless Group.

Goss S (1996) Bringing housing into community care. Journal of Interprofessional Care 10(3): 231–9.

Goss S, Kent C (1995) Health and Housing – Working Together? London: Joseph Rowntree Foundation/Policy Press.

Gove WR (Ed) (1982) Deviance and Mental Illness. In Sage Annual Reviews of Studies, Vol. 6: Deviance. London: Sage Publications.

Granger CV, Greer D (1976) Functional status measurement and medical rehabilitation outcomes. Archive of Physical Medical Rehabilitation 57: 103–9.

Greene JA (1979) Science, nursing and nursing science: a conceptual analysis. Advances in Nursing Science 2(1): 57–64.

Hales A, Magnus M (1991) Feeding the homeless. Journal of Nursing Administration 21(12): 36-41.

Hamid AW, McCarthy M (1989) Community psychiatric care for homeless people in Inner London. Health Trends 21(3): 67–9.

Hamilton D (1981) The Healers: A History of Medicine in Scotland. Edinburgh: Canongate.

Hart E (1991) Ghost in the machine. Health Service Journal (Dec 5): 20–2.

Health Visitors' Association/General Medical Services Committee (1989) Homeless Families and their Health. London: BMA Publications.

Heptinstall D (1989) Glimmer of Psychiatric Hope for Homeless Men in London. Social Work Today 20(24): 16–17.

Heuston J, Stern R, Stilwell B (1989) From the Margins to the Mainstream: Collaboration in Planning Services with Single Homeless People. London: Single Homeless Health Action Research Project/West Lambeth Health Authority.

Hirschi T, Gottfredson M (1983) Age and the explanation of crime. American Journal of Sociology 89: 552–84.

Hollander D, Hepplewhite R (1990) 'Mentally ill and nowhere to go' and 'No grounds for public fear. Community Care (802): 16–17.

Holmes C (1990) Alternatives to natural science foundations for nursing. International Journal of Nursing 27(3): 187–98.

Houghton P, Timperley N (1992) The Single European Market and the Implications for Public Housing. Birmingham: Birmingham City Council Housing Department, European Community.

Hudson B (1989) Down, out and neglected. Health Service Journal 99(5142): 334–5.

Hughes CP (1992) Community psychiatric nursing and depression in elderly people. Journal of Advanced Nursing 17: 34–42.

Hunt SM (1981) The development of quality of life profiles: the Nottingham health profile. In Berfenstam R, Jonsson E (Eds) Proceedings from the International Workshop on Quality of Life Measures, Methodology and Application in Health Policy, Uppsala, Sweden.

Hunt SM, McEwen J (1980) The development of a subjective health indicator. Sociology of Health and Illness 2(3): 232–46.

Ingram R (1991) Why does nursing need theory. Journal of Advanced Nursing 16: 350–3.

Jenkins R (1996) Social Identity. London: Routledge.

Jessop M (1987) Who should care for the health of the homeless? General Practitioner (Jan 9): 18.

Johnson L (1991) Callista Roy – an Adaptation Model. Newbury Park, CA: Sage.

Johnson M, Challis D for the Department of Health and Social Security (1983) The Realities and Potential of Community Care. In Elderly People and their Service Needs. London: HMSO, Ch. 6.

Julty S (1981) Men and their health – a strained alliance. M Magazine (Winter): 5–6.

Kaplan H (1991) Acorns and oaks, sowing and reaping ... and cabbages and kings. Featured essay on: Robins LN, Rutter M (1990) Straight and devious pathways from childhood to adulthood. Contemporary Sociology 20(1): 7–10.

Kelling K, Lawson P, McMillan I (1991) Homelessness. Nursing Times 87(48):26–32.

Keyes S, Kennedy M (1992) Sick to Death of Homelessness – an Investigation into the Links between Homelessness, Health and Mortality. London: CRISIS at Christmas.

Khan RL, Goldfarb AS, Pollack M, Peck A (1960) Brief objective measures for the determination of mental status in the aged. American Journal of Psychiatry 117: 326–8.

Kitching R (1991) Poverty and Deprivation in Hammersmith and Fulham. Research Report. London: London Borough of Hammersmith and Fulham Development Planning Department.

Kitsuse (1968) In Spitzer SP, Denzin NK (Eds) The Mental Patient – Studies in the Sociology of Deviance. London: McGraw-Hill.

Knight BJ, Osborn SG, West D (1977) Early marriage and criminal tendency in males. British Journal of Criminology 17: 348–60.

Laing I (1993) Single Homelessness and Mental Health Issues in Glasgow. Glasgow: Glasgow City Housing/Richmond Fellowship.

Lamb HR, Talbot JA (1986) The homeless mentally ill: the perspective of the American Psychiatric Association. Journal of the American Medical Association 256(4): 498–501.

Leather P, Kirk H (1991) Age File: The Facts. Oxford: Anchor Housing Association.

Leddington S, Shiner P (1991) Sometimes it makes you frightened to go to hospital ... they treat you like dirt. Health Service Journal 101(5277): 2124.

Lewis J (1993) Collaborative planning. Journal of Interprofessional Care 7(1): 7–14.

Lovell B (1986) Health visiting and homeless families. Health Visitor 59(11): 334-7.

Lowry S (1991) Housing and Health. London: BMJ Publications.

McAndrew L, Hanley J (1988) Survey of the Younger Disabled in the Community in Lothian. Rehabilitation Studies Unit Research Project. Edinburgh: University of Edinburgh.

McDonald DD (1986) Health care and cost containment for the homeless: curricular implications. Journal of Nursing Education 25(6): 261–4.

McIntosh J (1985) District nursing: a case of political marginality. In White R (Ed) Political Issues in Nursing, Vol. 1. Chichester: John Wiley and Sons, Ch. 3.

McKenna SP, Hunt SM, McEwen J (1981) Weighting the seriousness of perceived health problems using Thurstone's method of paired comparisons. International Journal of Epidemiology 10(1): 93–7.

Mackenzie AE (1992) Learning from experience in the community: an ethnographic study of district nurse students. Journal of Advanced Nursing 17: 682–91.

Macmillan D, Miller H, Wormesley J (1992) Homelessness and Health – a Needs Assessment in the Greater Glasgow Health Board Area. Glasgow: Greater Glasgow Health Board Health Information Unit.

McMillan I (1991) Barred from treatment. Nursing Times 87(48): 23.

Mahoney Fl, Barthel DW (1965) Functional education: the Barthel index. Rehabilitation 22(23): 61–5.

Maslow A H (1943) A theory of human motivation. Psychological Review. No 50 pp 370-396.

Masters B Burke (1988) The nurse practitioner's surgery. Self Health (18): 22–3.

Means R (1996) Housing and community care for older people – joint working at the local level. Journal of Interprofessional Care 10(3): 273.

Medical Campaign Project (1990) Good Practice on Discharge of Single Homeless People with Particular Reference to Mental Health Units. London: MCP.

Medical Campaign Project/Campaign for Homeless and Rootless (1991) Newsletter on Mental Health and Homelessness. London: MCP/CHAR.

Metters J and the Department of Health (1991) Health care for the homeless and rootless – A view from central government. Journal of the Royal Society of Health 111(92): 75–7.

Morfett R, Pidgeon J (1991) Mental health: unity in action. Social Work Today 22(17): 16–17.

Murdoch I (1992) Metaphysics as a Guide to Morals. London: Penguin.

Murie A (1988) Housing, homelessness and social work. In Becker S, MacPherson S (Eds) Public Issues, Private Pain: Poverty, Social Work and Social Policy. London: Social Services/Insight Books, p 283.

National Council for Voluntary Organisations (1988) Time To Act on Community Care: NCVO'S Response to Sir Roy Griffiths' Report: 'Community Care: Agenda for Action'. London: NCVO.

Nelson S, Kirk D (1991) Excluding Youth: Poverty among Young People Living away from Home. Edinburgh: Bridges Project.

Norman I, Parker F (1990) Psychiatric patients' views of their lives before and after moving to a hostel: a qualitative study. Journal of Advanced Nursing (15): 1036–44.

Norman IJ, Redfern SJ, Tomalin DA, Oliver S (1992) Developing Flanagan's critical incident technique to elicit indicators of high and low quality nursing care from patients and their nurses. Journal of Advanced Nursing (17): 590–600.

O'Meachair G, Burns A (1988) Irish Homelessness. The Hidden Dimension: A Strategy for Change. London: City of Westminster CARA.

Onyett S (1989) Sweeping up Homelessness in New York. Openmind 41: 10–11.

Oppenheim C (1991) Poverty in London: An Overview. London: Child Poverty Action Group.

Orem D (1995) Nursing: concepts of practice. 5th edition. London: Mosby.

Park PB (1989) Health Care for the Homeless. Clinical Nurse Specialist 3(4): 171–5.

Patton MQ (1990) Qualitative Evaluation and Research Methods. Newbury Park, CA: Sage.

Peterken L (1990) General management in Glasgow – the search for efficiency. Health Services Management Journal (Oct): 216–20.

Phillips J (1977) Nursing systems and nursing models. Image 9(1): 4–7.

Platt S (1988) Standards or choice? New Society 83(1319): 14–15.

Porter R (Ed) (1990) The Faber Book of Madness. London: Faber.

Powell PV (1987a) The use of an accident and emergency department by the single homeless. Health Bulletin 45(5): 255–62.

Powell PV (1987b) A house doctor scheme for primary health care for single homeless in Edinburgh. Journal of the Royal College of General Practitioners 37(303): 444–7.

Powell PV (1988) Qualitative assessment in the evaluation of the Edinburgh primary health care scheme for single homeless hostel dwellers. Community Medicine 10(3): 185–96.

Quick R (1990) Lost in America. Nursing Times 86(30): 44–7.

Rapport B (1981) Helping men ask for help. M Magazine (Winter): 3–27.

Rapport N (1993) Diverse World Views in an English Village. Edinburgh: Edinburgh University Press.

Redhead S (1984) Deviance and the law. In Abrams P, Brown R (Eds) UK Society: Work, Urbanism and Inequality. London: Weidenfield and Nicolson, p 294.

Reed J, Robbins I (1991) Models of nursing: their relevance to the care of elderly people. Journal of Advanced Nursing 16: 1350–7.

Rickford F, Montague A (1987) The travellers tales. New Society: Race and Society Section (Dec 4): 2–3.

Robins Lee, N and Rutter M (Eds) (1990) Straight and Devious Pathways from Childhood to Adulthood. Cambridge: Cambridge University Press.

Rock P, McIntosh M (1974) Deviance and Social Control. London: Tavistock Publications.

Roper A, Logan WW, Tierney A (1990) The Elements of Nursing: A Model for Nursing Based on a Model of Living. 3rd Edn. Edinburgh: Churchill Livingstone.

Ross F (1993) Editorial. Journal of Interprofessional Care 7(1): 6.

Roth JA (1963) Timetables. Indianapolis: Bobbs-Merrill.

Roy C (1977) Decision-making by the Physically Ill and Adaptation During Illness. Unpublished dissertation, Library of University of California at Los Angeles USA.

Roy C (1980) The Roy adaptation model. In Riehl JP, Roy C (Eds) Conceptual Models for Nursing Practice. Norwalk, CT: Appleton-Century-Crofts.

Roy C (1988) An explication of the philosophical assumptions of the Roy adaptation model. Nursing Science quarterly 1(1): 26–34.

Roy C, Andrews HA (1991) The Roy Adaptation Model – The definitive statement. Appleton and Lange USA.

Royal College of Physicians/British Geriatrics Society (1992) Standardised Assessment Scales for Elderly People. Report of Joint Workshops of the Research Unit of the Royal College of Physicians and the British Geriatrics Society. London: RCP/BGR.

Runciman P (1989) Health assessment of the elderly at home: the case for shared learning. Journal of Advanced Nursing (14): 111–19.

Sampson RJ, Laub JH (1990) Crime and deviance over the life course: the salience of adult social bonds. American Sociological Review 55: 609–27.

Sanders C (1990) Homesick. New Statesman Society 3(88): 10–11.

Sarvimaki A (1988) Nursing as a moral, practical, communicative and creative activity. Journal of Advanced Nursing 13: 462–7.

Scottish Home and Health Department (1990) A Strategy for Nursing, Midwifery and Health Visiting in Scotland. Scotland: HMSO.

Shanks N (1981) Consistency of data collected from inmates of a common lodging house. Journal of Epidemiological Community Health 35: 153–5.

Shanks N, Smith SJ (1992) British public policy and the health of homeless people. Policy and Politics 20(1): 35–46.

Shelter (1988) Britain's Housing Crisis: The Facts and Figures. London: Shelter.

Shelter (1990a) Progress Report. London: Shelter.

Shelter (1990b) Homelessness in England: The Facts. London: Shelter.

Shelter (1991) Homelessness - What's the Problem? London: Shelter.

Simon Community (1989) Time for a National Response to the Homeless Crisis. Dublin: Simon Community.

Single Homeless in London (1987) Report of the SHIL. London: SHIL.

Single Homeless in London (1989) High Care Housing: Providing Housing, Support and Personal Care for Homeless People with Special Needs in London. Twickenham: SHIL.

Sintonen H (1981) An approach to measuring and valuing health states. Social Science in Medicine 15C: 55–65.

Skinner HA (1982) Drug and Alcohol Questionnaires. Addiction Research Foundation, 33 Russell Street, Toronto, Canada.

Smart A (1988) Villages of Glasgow, Vol. 1. Edinburgh: John Donald Publishers.

Smith C (1989) Closing the Door - Changes to Benefits for Hostel Residents after October. London: Shelter.

Smith JP (1981) Sociology and Nursing. 2nd Edn. Edinburgh: Churchill Livingstone.

Snaith RP (1991) Measurement in psychiatry. British Journal of Psychiatry 157P: 78-82.

Snaith RP (1992) Anhedonia: exclusion from the pleasure dome – a useful marker of biological depression. British Medical Journal 305: 134.

Spitzer SP, Denzin NK (1968) The Mental Patient – Studies in the Sociology of Deviance. London: McGraw-Hill Book Co.

Statistical Package for the Social Sciences (1990) SPSS Inc, Wacker Drive, Chicago, Illinois 60606, USA.

Stephenson C (1991) The concept of hope revisited for nursing. Journal of Advanced Nursing 16: 1456–61.

Stern R (1990) Working for (some) patients. Roof 15(1): 18–19.

Stern R, Stillwell B (1989) From margin to mainstream. Health Service Journal 99 (5169).

Stilwell B, Stern R (1989) Treadmill on trial. Health Service Journal 99(5167): 1102–3.

Streetly A (1987) Health care for travellers: one year's experience. British Medical Journal 294: 492–4.

Taylor I (1992) Discharged with Care – a Report on Practical Arrangements for People Leaving Psychiatric Hospital and the Prevention of Homelessness. Edinburgh: Lothian Health Board Mental Health Unit/Scottish Council for Single Homeless.

Thomas E (1991) Unstable lodgings. Nursing Times 87(30): 42–4.

Thompson R, Atkinson J (1989) Homelessness and health. Nursing Standard 3(48): 30–2.

Timms PW, Fry AH (1989) Homelessness and health. Health Trends 21(3): 70–1.

Toon PD, Thomas K, Doherty M (1987) Audit of work at a medical centre for the homeless over one year. Journal of the Royal College of General Practitioners 37(296): 120–2.

Victor CR, Connelly J, Roderick P, Cohen C (1989) Use of hospital services by homeless families in an Inner London health district. British Medical Journal 299: 725–7.

Victoria Community Health Council (1984) Falling Through the Net: A Report on Health Care for Homeless People and Hostel Dwellers in the Victoria Health Authority. Victoria Community Health Council.

Wall P (1991) Health and homelessness. Health Service Journal 101(5247): 16–17.

Wake M (1991) Housing and Care Needs of Older Homeless People. London: London Borough of Camden Social Services Department.

Watson S, Austerberry H (1986) Housing and Homelessness: A Feminist Perspective. London: Routledge and Kegan Paul.

Weller MPI, Weller BGA (1988) Mental illness and social policy. Medicine Science and the Law 28(1): 47–53.

Whetstone WR, Reid JC (1991) Health promotion of older adults: perceived barriers. Journal of Advanced Nursing 16: 1343–9.

Whynes DK (1990) Reported health problems and the socio-economic characteristics of the single homeless. British Journal of Social Work 20(4): 355–64.

Williams RP (1987) Achieving co-operation. Housing Review 36(2): 66–8.

Williams S, Allen L (1989) Health Care for Single Homeless People. London: Policy Studies Institute.

Win JK, Cooper JE, Surtonus N (1974) Measurement and Classification of Psychiatric Symptoms. In Present State Examination. Cambridge: Cambridge University Press, p 141–87.

Wooton H (1985) A new year – but little year for the single homeless. Health and Social Service Journal 95(4978): 1564–5.

World Health Organization (1989) Health Principles of Housing. Geneva: WHO.

Worth A, McIntosh J, Carney O, Lugton J (1995) Assessment of Need for District Nursing. Department of Nursing and Community Health. Glasgow: Glasgow Caledonian University.

Yeudall J (1988) The Medical Campaign Project: Campaign for Improved Access to Health Care for Single Homeless People: Final Report. London: MCP.

Zigmond AS, Snaith RP (1983) The hospital anxiety and depression scale. Acta Psychiatrica Scandinavica 67: 361–70.

Index